GW00696841

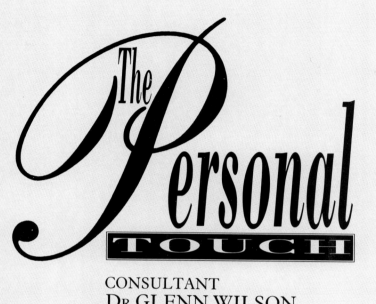

The Personal Touch

CONSULTANT
Dr GLENN WILSON

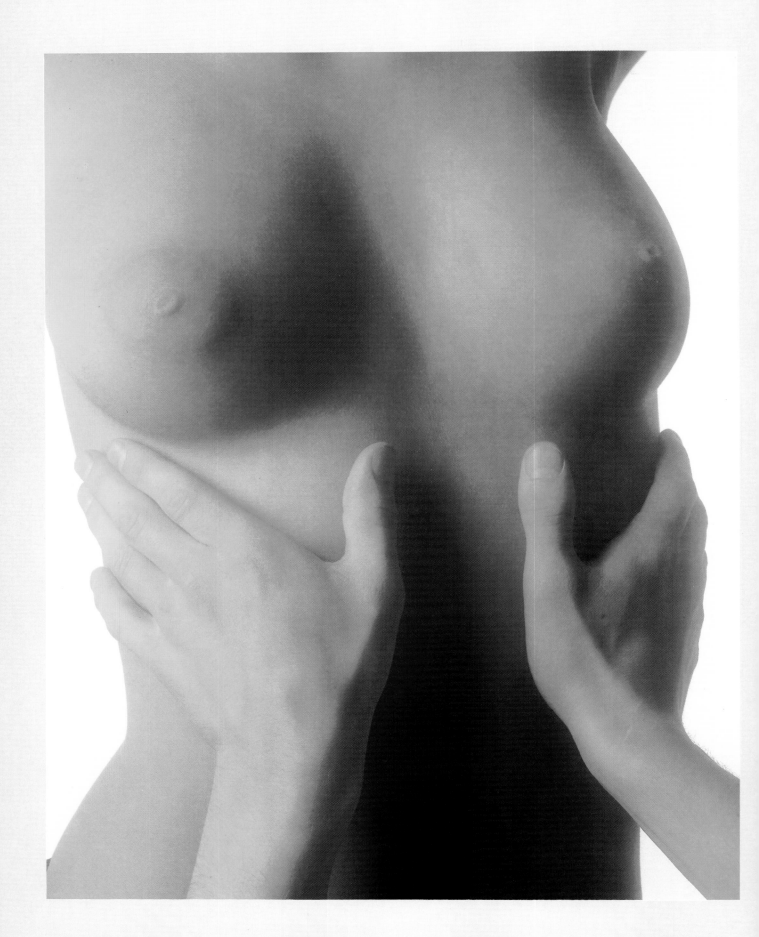

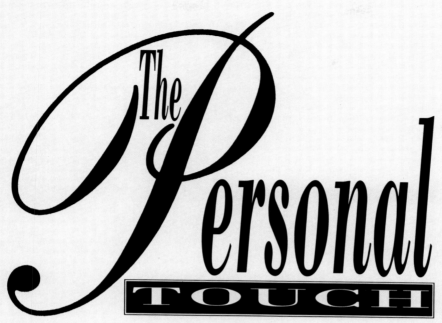

The Personal Touch

CONSULTANT
Dr GLENN WILSON

Macdonald Illustrated

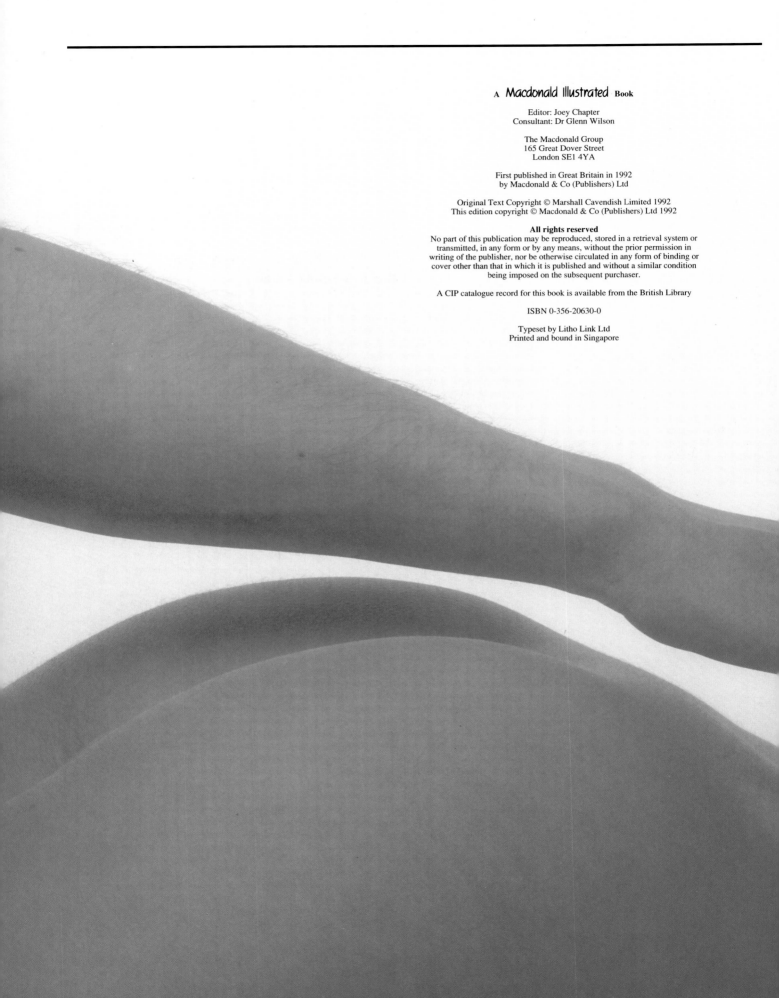

A Macdonald Illustrated Book

Editor: Joey Chapter
Consultant: Dr Glenn Wilson

The Macdonald Group
165 Great Dover Street
London SE1 4YA

First published in Great Britain in 1992
by Macdonald & Co (Publishers) Ltd

Original Text Copyright © Marshall Cavendish Limited 1992
This edition copyright © Macdonald & Co (Publishers) Ltd 1992

All rights reserved
No part of this publication may be reproduced, stored in a retrieval system or
transmitted, in any form or by any means, without the prior permission in
writing of the publisher, nor be otherwise circulated in any form of binding or
cover other than that in which it is published and without a similar condition
being imposed on the subsequent purchaser.

A CIP catalogue record for this book is available from the British Library

ISBN 0-356-20630-0

Typeset by Litho Link Ltd
Printed and bound in Singapore

CONTENTS

INTRODUCTION 6

SETTING THE SCENE

A TIME AND PLACE FOR LOVING 10
CREATING BETTER CONDITIONS FOR SEX ... 18
DRESSING FOR SEX 24
BREASTS AND SEX 30
FEMALE FANTASIES 36
MALE FANTASIES 42

CREATIVE LOVEMAKING

MAKING SEX MORE MEMORABLE 50
TOWARDS ORGASM 58
COME TOGETHER 66
ORAL SEX 74
IMAGINATIVE SEX 82
SEX AND MOVEMENT 90

HOW TO SEDUCE YOUR WIFE 96
HOW TO SEDUCE YOUR HUSBAND 106
MORE ROMANTIC LOVEMAKING 114
IMPROVE YOUR ORGASMS 122

A DASH OF SPICE

SEX AIDS 132
MAKING A SEXY VIDEO 140
FETISHISM 148
GROUP SEX FANTASIES 153
WHEN THINGS GO WRONG 158
REVIVING YOUR SEX LIFE 164
A LIFETIME OF LOVING 170
CONTRACEPTION 176
SEXUAL DISEASES 182
AIDS 186

INDEX 190
ACKNOWLEDGEMENTS 192

Although the artworks in this book do not depict men wearing condoms, we do recommend the use of them, especially in a new relationship, or where you have not known your partner very long.

INTRODUCTION

In a good sexual relationship, the mind is involved just as much as the body. Lovemaking is a time when we can indulge in our wildest fantasies, step beyond our usual boundaries, and explore the most hidden aspects of our personalities. For the loving and receptive couple who wish to share in each other's sexuality, exploring fantasy and enjoying being inventive and adventurous can be an extremely rich and rewarding experience.

For most happily established couples, lovemaking tends to fall into a routine – one of the usual few positions, preceded by tried and tested caresses. There is absolutely nothing wrong with this – it makes sense to stick with what you know suits you both when you want to be sure of sexual fulfilment.

But there are occasions – especially when a relationship has lasted a long time – when it is well worth trying something new, for experimenting and being creative can add new experiences and sensations to even the best of lovemaking. It may be something as

simple as a new lovemaking position, or as daring as acting out your sexual fantasies. But it will bring a new excitement and novelty to your sex life, and you will both feel richer for it.

Never be afraid to try something new – as long as you both want to try it. Coercion is not part of any good relationship. Suggestion, however, is – and you may well find that, if you suggest something a little different to your partner, he or she may well have been thinking along the same lines. Being open-minded at all times is after all one of the keystones of a successful and progressive partnership.

The most important thing is to *share*. Sex is the

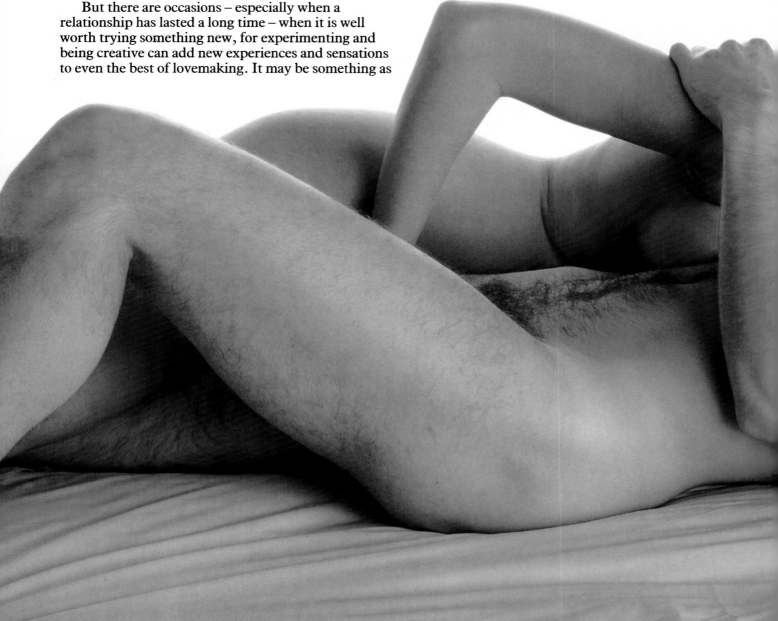

most intimate expression of sharing a couple can experience; but often the sharing is not extended beyond this horizon. It is not just bodies that should merge: share your innermost fears, fantasies and desires, and you will not only learn more about your partner as a complete person, but you will also grow to learn more about yourself. It takes trust – but then, this book is intended for couples who have a commitment to each other, and are therefore held together by bonds of mutual love and trust. A relationship where you need have no fear of opening up your soul will go a long way to ensuring a marvellous and fulfilling sex life.

Every relationship is different. What one couple enjoys, another might not. There are no rules. These are merely guidelines and suggestions, to encourage you to use your own resources of fantasy and widen your own personal horizons. Be guided by what feels good, and you will be assured of physical and emotional rewards for you both.

And remember – the best aid for wonderful sex cannot be bought in a shop or acquired from reading a book. All that is required is a sensitive and loving partner – and a little imagination . . .

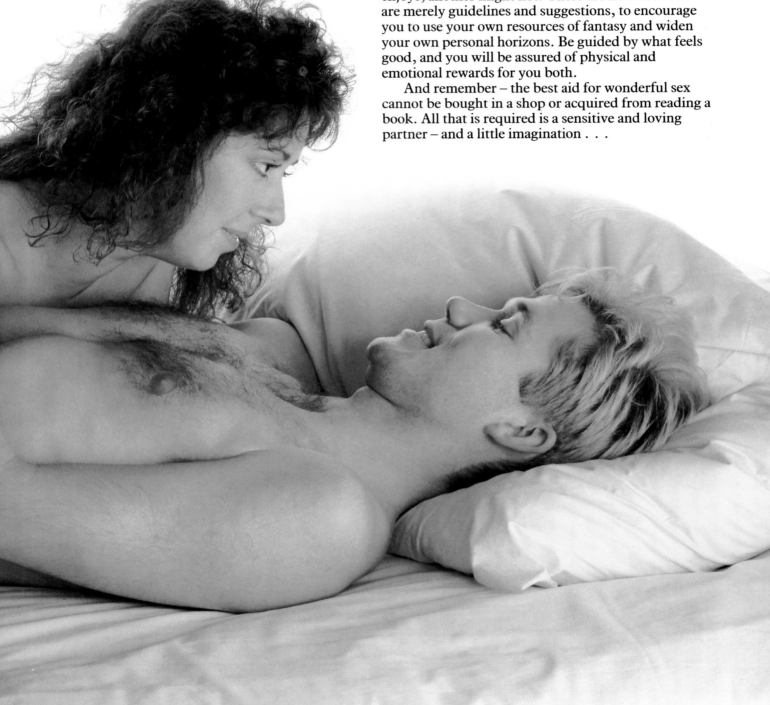

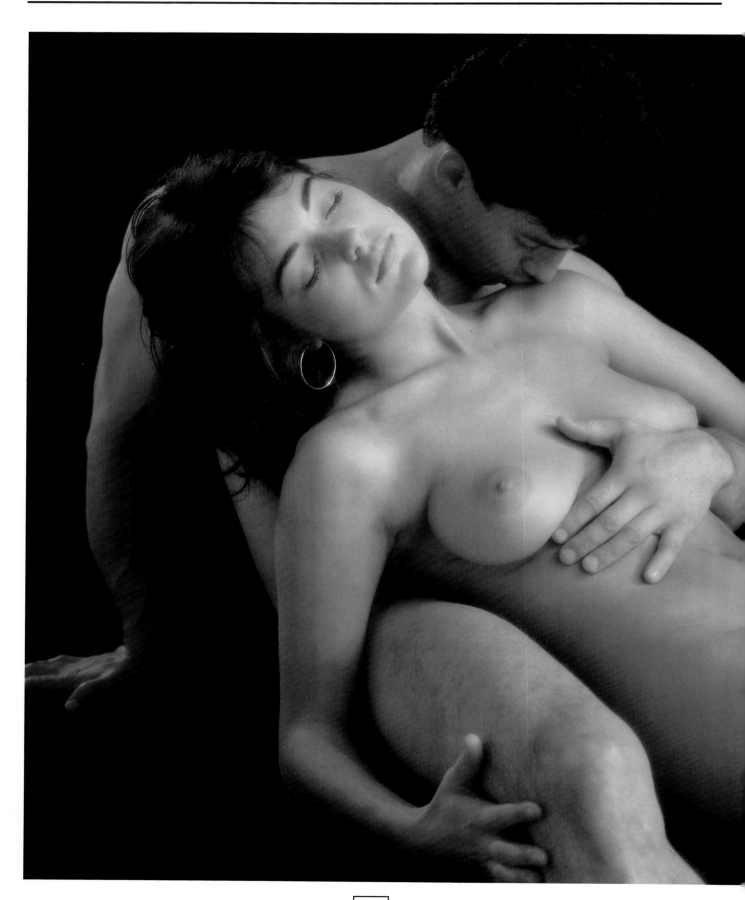

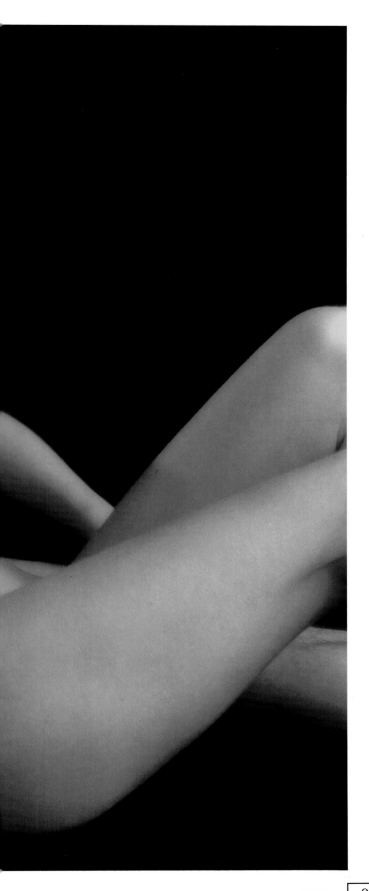

SETTING THE SCENE

You can make love at any time, virtually anywhere; but by ensuring that your surroundings, bodies and minds are in the right mood, you will bring untold benefits to your lovemaking. Take a little time and trouble to establish the best conditions for great sex, and experience the difference in your sensations and responses that results

A TIME AND PLACE FOR LOVING

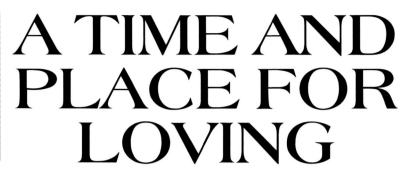

Like many things in life, a couple can tend to take sex for granted and accept a routine simply out of laziness. But there is really no reason for this to happen with loving and compatible partners

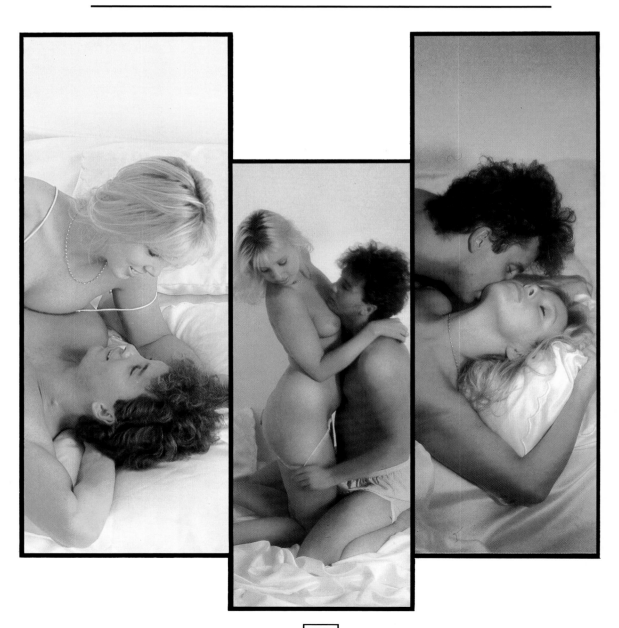

At the beginning of a sexual relationship, a couple will experiment extensively – exploring each other's bodies to discover what pleases each partner best, trying out different lovemaking positions until they settle on the one that brings the most satisfaction for both of them and, in their time apart, thinking of the pleasures of sexual moments that help strengthen the emotional bonds of the relationship.

After a while a couple usually settle down to a steady, but varied, sex life. However, 'steady' can soon turn into boring, and 'varied' into predictable.

It is all too easy to relegate sex to a lower position on the list of 'things to do'. Obviously worries about money, work and sundry other facets of our lives can temporarily preoccupy us, but if domestic trivia impinges on our sex lives, it can cause problems for the relationship.

EARLY TO BED, EARLY TO RISE

Many people feel at their sexiest in the morning, this applies in particular to men, who often wake up with an erection. Add to this the relaxed feeling from sleeping well and the intimate contact of being together for a few hours, and you have very conducive conditions for making love.

Too often, however, these times are lost – except perhaps on Saturday and Sunday – because making love with one eye on the clock or worrying about missing a train or bus is never going to be satisfying. There are, however, several solutions to overcoming the obstructions of your daily routine.

First, and perhaps most obvious, is to go to bed early occasionally. Sacrificing the late-night weather forecast can quickly pay dividends in your personal life. Too many people expect a quality sex life without creating the necessary conditions.

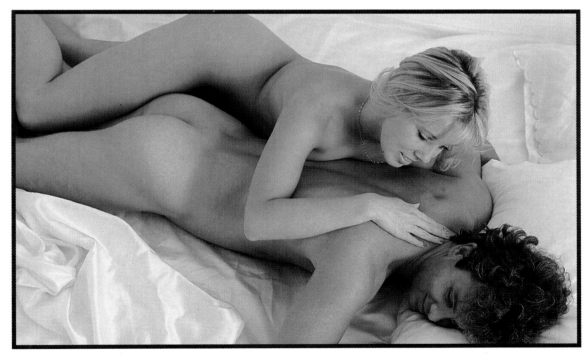

Waking up to a sensual massage is one of the best ways to start the day – wait until your partner is half awake before moving to the more erogenous zones of the body

FIND THE TIME

The first thing to do is to find the time to make love. Clinical experience suggests that the majority of couples make love at 10 o'clock on a Friday night, in their bed. While there is nothing implicitly wrong in making love before you go to sleep – and a bed is therefore the ideal location – if lovemaking just becomes another regular 'job' to be done, rather like the weekly shopping or cleaning the car, prospects for a happy and fulfilling sex life are not always the best that they could be.

If one or both of you work every day, then making love during weekdays is more difficult than at weekends. But for lovers who are in tune with each other's sexuality, it is surprising how much can be fitted into a busy routine if the desire to do so is there.

START THE DAY RIGHT

If you wake early, you will be able to find the time to relax in bed rather than having to scramble around dressing and breakfasting; it is surprising how quickly sex appears on the morning menu.

Being woken gently by a loving partner with some sensual massage can be an exquisite experience for both men and women. If you are the first awake, begin gently and sensitively exploring your partner's body. Cuddle up close and kiss them gently. Stroke their face, neck and shoulders. Keep this up and they are half awake before moving on to the more erogenous zones of the body.

This is not a time to be selfish. Wait until they are fully aroused and wanting to make love before you try for full intercourse. On some occasions, you may not

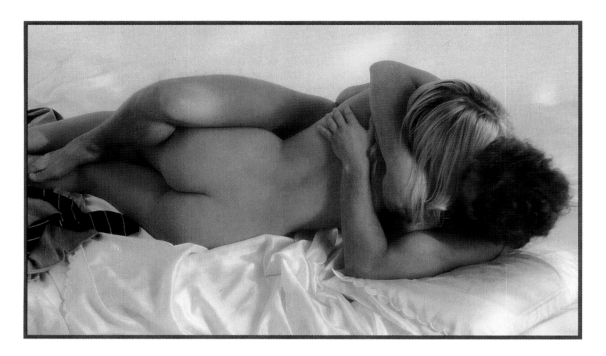

(right) On a warm day, a secluded conservatory can be an ideal venue for lovemaking – in this position, penetration is very deep and the couple can caress and kiss

(left) Spending time together in bed, especially during the day, can add an air of intimacy to a loving relationship, even when you are not making love

want to do this. If the time and the mood are right, continue to use your hands and mouth to increase the tempo and bring your partner to orgasm in the way they like best. Your time will come another morning.

Another solution to fitting in early morning sex is 'quickies'. These do not have to be confined to the bed, or even the bedroom.

If your morning routine involves a shower or a bath, then there is every reason for doing it together. Washing and soaping each other is an extremely sensual form of foreplay for virtually everyone. Whether you want to make love during or after is entirely a matter of personal preference, and again it is not necessary to aim for penis-in-vagina sex. Oral sex is often one of the quickest ways to bring your partner to orgasm, and the knowledge that both of you have clean genitals makes after a bath the time that many people are able to feel most at ease.

DRESSING AND UNDRESSING
While you are dressing can also be an exciting time. If you are in the mood, it is very easy to turn the simple act of dressing into a sexy striptease. Research into human sexuality has shown conclusively that men are more easily turned on by visual displays of sex than women are, so it is probably a more effective tactic for a woman.

Rather than quickly jumping into your clothes, dress slowly – perhaps walking about the bedroom naked or part-naked for some of the time. Try dressing your bottom and top halves separately, rather than putting on your bra and panties first. A glimpse of naked breasts being covered last, or exposing your vulva as you bend down to choose some clothes can often turn your partner on to the idea of a quickie.

Even if you do not make love in the mornings,

loving and considerate behaviour, extending to gentle foreplay, will at least hint at what is to come later in the evening.

AFTERNOON DELIGHT
Making love at lunchtime or in the afternoon, is something that most people reserve for the weekends. Medical research has shown, however that the male sex hormone that is present in both sexes peaks at 3.00 in the afternoon, regardless of when you may have woken up, which suggests that the afternoon should be a very sexy time.

If you work close to home, there is no reason not to plan the occasional sexy lunchtime. For some couples, because the whole idea is thought of as slightly 'naughty', these adventures are a great turn-on. If you wish, you can also turn it into a kind of fantasy game – pretending that you are having an affair and having sex in secret.

But, as with all things in life, spontaneity can add much to an episode of lovemaking. If you see each other for lunch, or it is not particularly difficult for you both to be at home, an early morning telephone call to suggest the idea may be very welcome. Just a hint such as 'Can I see you for lunch at home, I've got something very special for you' should be enough to set the scene of what is to come.

If you want, you can take it a stage further by organizing some of your favourite food and perhaps some wine or champagne.

If you do not live close to work, afternoon love-making may have to wait for Saturday and Sunday. Few people can find the money, or face the faint embarrassment, of booking into a hotel during the day. But the occasional half-day holiday may be worth taking if you both feel like it.

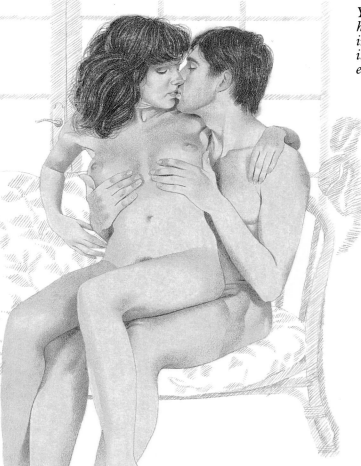

You need not go up the stairs to bed to make love – stop halfway there and you have a perfect venue for intercourse in a standing position. Leave on a couple of items of clothing – stockings and suspenders – and add extra excitement

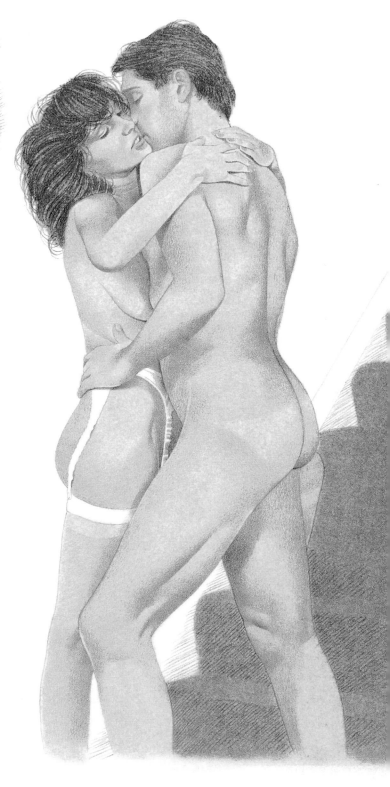

SOME ENCHANTED EVENING

While the evenings are regarded as 'own time' by most people, it is surprising how crowded they can be. Added to a domestic routine of washing, ironing, cleaning and cooking is, for most people, a 'social' routine that can leave little time left for lovemaking. In addition to lack of time, tiredness can dull the edge of anyone's sexual appetite.

Again, it is up to both of you to make the time to spend together, if only to talk to each other intimately. If every evening is taken up with domestic chores or socializing, it is not difficult for sex to be relegated to Sunday mornings only.

This kind of lifestyle can soon take over a relationship fairly early on and sow the seeds of difficulty in the long term.

Obviously, demanding that your partner stops doing something that he or she enjoys is not a satisfactory answer. But if you do find that you rarely have time to communicate about your needs and feelings, you will probably find you never have the time to express them either.

There are no pre-set rules about when to make love. There is no biological reason for not making love at any time of the day. The only restriction is time and

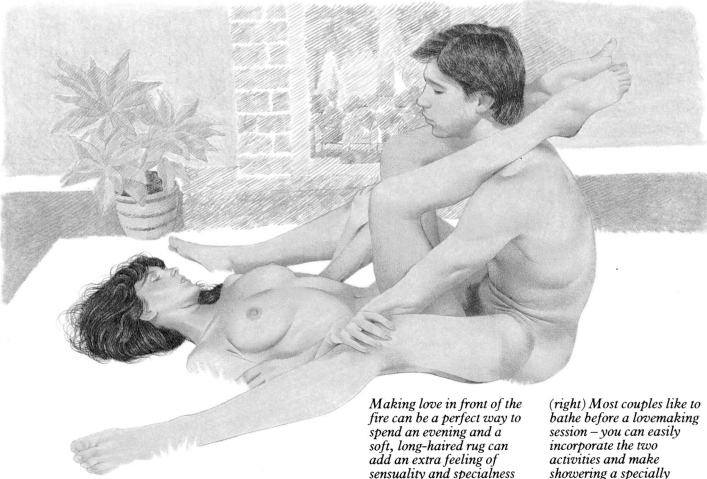

Making love in front of the fire can be a perfect way to spend an evening and a soft, long-haired rug can add an extra feeling of sensuality and specialness to the occasion

(right) Most couples like to bathe before a lovemaking session – you can easily incorporate the two activities and make showering a specially sensuous part of foreplay

it is up to each loving couple to find that time and not let sex become a low priority in life in general.

UPSTAIRS/ DOWNSTAIRS

Although most couples make love most of the time in bed, any home provides a variety of venues for love-making, if only occasionally to add some variation and fun to a full and satisfying relationship.

For 'quickies' virtually anywhere is suitable, but for longer bouts of lovemaking warmth and comfort are essential. Making love on the bathroom floor after a bath can be exciting, but cold, hard floor coverings can soon dampen passions and freeze out enjoyment.

Alternatively, if an evening at home spent listening to music or watching television naturally leads to sex, breaking off to adjourn to the bedroom may not be a good idea if the sofa or the carpet in front of the fire is just as comfortable and helps to preserve the mood of the moment.

THE WHOLE HOUSE
If you live in a house, downstairs probably provides you with a kitchen, lounge and perhaps a separate dining room. By their functional nature each room will provide you with different furniture and furnishings that can be used in your lovemaking.

THE LOUNGE
Most lounges are furnished with a sofa which, if it is long enough and firm enough, provides an excellent place to make love. One with a drop-down end, or a chaise longue can be even better and have certain advantages over a bed.

For rear entry, a sofa creates many possibilities and variations, all of which provide deep penetration.
☐ The woman kneels on the sofa, facing one of the ends. She leans forward and rests her forearms on the side of the sofa. The man kneels behind her and enters her vagina. This has the advantage of allowing the woman to support her weight so the position is not too tiring and she is also able to move backwards and forwards and control the angle and depth of penetration. The man can reach round to fondle her breasts and caress her clitoris.

☐ The woman kneels on the sofa, facing the back, and supports herself on the back. The man stands behind her and inserts his penis. The man's movements are somewhat restricted and he will probably need to keep his balance by holding the woman's thighs. He can draw her towards him, and push her away, or she can control the movements.

☐ The woman kneels on the floor with as much of her body flat on the sofa as possible. The man kneels on the floor behind her and holds on to her sides. Movement is fairly restricted, but this position is less tiring than the unsupported 'doggie' position.

☐ The woman leans over the side or back of the sofa and the man stands behind her and holds on to her sides. The woman has very little control, but penetration can be exceedingly deep.

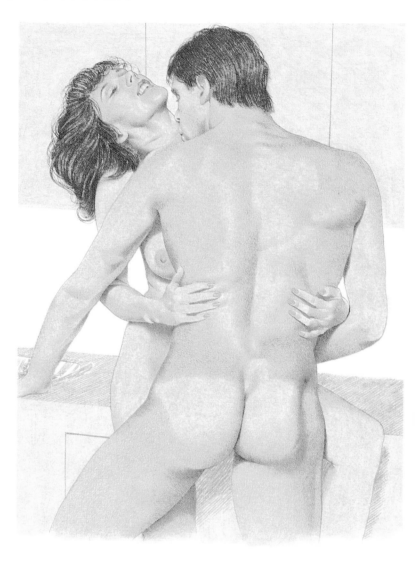

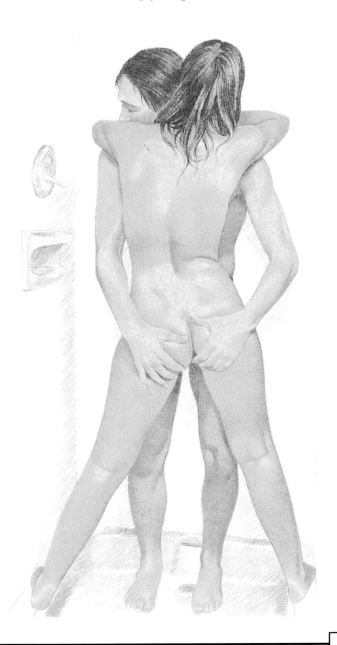

The kitchen need not be reserved just for cooking – it can also be a perfect place for lovemaking whether it is first thing in the morning or late at night

FACE-TO-FACE

If the sofa is long enough, all man-on-top positions are possible. But as with the rear-entry positions the height and level of the sofa can be used for some variations, depending on what positions they prefer to make love in.

☐ The woman sits with her bottom on the edge of the sofa. The man kneels in between her thighs and inserts his penis. His hands are free to fondle her breasts and if he leans back he has a good view of his penis entering her vagina. Movement is almost completely under the man's control, but the woman can move from side to side.

☐ A variation of this position is for the woman to wrap her legs around the man's neck. This restricts movement further but can produce novel sensations by varying the angle of entry and allowing the man greater depth of penetration.

ARE YOU SITTING COMFORTABLY?

If you do want to combine making love with watching your favourite television programme or video, there is no need to move the TV set to the bedroom. The versatility of the sofa provides the answer. There are two basic rear-entry positions, both of which can be held comfortably for some time but the variations are infinite. Spend time experimenting with your partner to see what turns you on most.

☐ The man sits on the edge of the sofa and the woman lowers herself onto his penis, facing away from him. His hands are free to caress her breasts and stimulate her clitoris.

☐ The 'spoons' position is also suitable, but the man may have to prop himself up on his elbow.

THE FLOOR

The lounge floor provides a firm base for lovemaking, and its firmness may create some advantages over the bed or the sofa. However, carpets of harsh material or a high synthetic fibre content can be uncomfortable, causing abrasions and skin burns.

Any other piece of furniture, such as a small footstool or pouffe can easily be employed in ways that you find suitable. It is up to you both to find out the best things for you. Be imaginative, and you may be pleasantly surprised.

THE KITCHEN

Not a room which most people particularly associate with romance, the kitchen is nonetheless one in which we spend a great deal of time. While the modern-day kitchen table may be neither large nor firm enough for lovemaking, the image of 'quickie' sex still has its place within the kitchen's confines.

Most work surfaces and appliances are built at such a level that they display the buttocks at a very provocative angle. While sex over the hob is obviously dangerous, most areas of the kitchen can provide excellent support for a standing rear-entry quickie.

GOING UP

For standing positions it is best – for reasons of anatomy – that the woman is higher than the man. Standing on a small stool, or even a stable pile of telephone directories, is perfectly adequate providing that you have some means of support such as a wall.

If you have stairs in the house they provide a

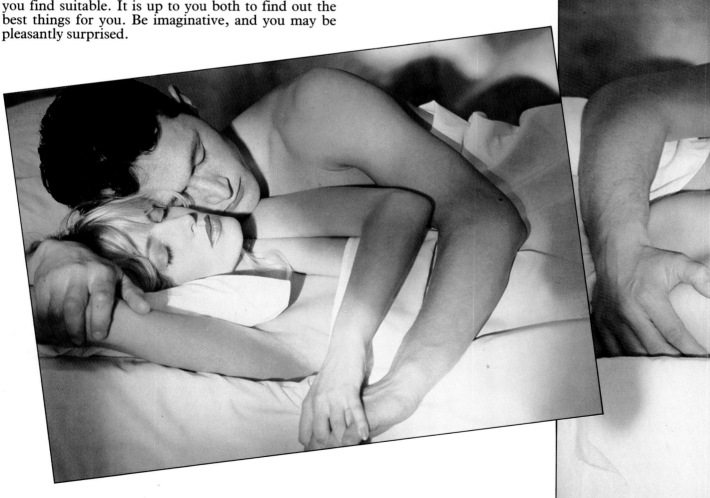

ready-made and stable prop. As long as the woman stands on one step above the man almost any part of the flight of stairs is suitable. But make sure you do not overbalance.

THE BATHROOM

Bathing or showering together is a very sensual experience. Unfortunately, the average bath is not usually large enough to make love in. Even if they are long enough, and one partner can put up with the taps, they are not really wide enough to allow for many different positions. There are some that are possible without one partner being in danger of drowning, but man-on-top positions can be difficult to achieve with both safety and satisfaction.

☐ Depending on the length of your bath, rear entry is possible to different degrees. The most suitable is a doggie position where the woman raises her buttocks out of the water and the man enters her by kneeling behind.

☐ The man lies back and rests on his elbows. The woman sits astride him and leans back, supporting herself on his knees. She can then place her legs over his shoulders. Movement is restricted, but the feeling of 'weightlessness' given by the water adds an extra dimension.

Showers, by their design, restrict lovemaking to mostly standing positions. They are, however, many couples' favourite place for oral sex. For both men and women, the active partner kneels on the shower floor with their head level with the other's penis or vulva, while the passive partner remains standing.

A ROOM FOR LOVING

For the truly loving and adventurous couple there are absolutely no restrictions on where and when they make love. Each partnership is unique, emotionally and sexually, and by experimenting and continually adding to your repertoire of lovemaking times and places, you can only enrich your relationship.

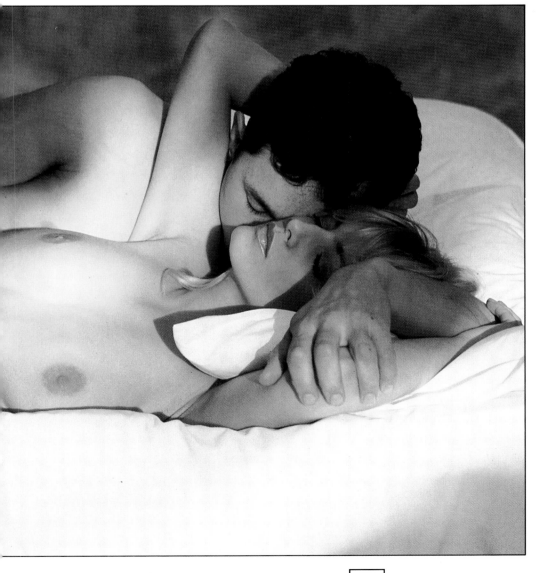

Making love during the day, when neither partner is tired, means that once you have climaxed you can spend time lying close before starting again – as with most things, the more time you have, the better

CREATING BETTER CONDITIONS FOR SEX

To get the best out of your sex life, you need to invest time and effort – for just as in anything else, a little extra work will bring its own rewards

Creating the best conditions for sex is often a problem for many couples and much of the time their lovemaking is not as enjoyable as it should be. With a little more thought and preparation, however, sex could be made much more relaxing and fulfilling.

As well as the various psychological and emotional preparations that could make things better, there are also a number of practical steps they can take to improve their lovelife.

MAKE MORE TIME
One of the worst enemies of a good sex life is time. Many couples relegate sex, and indeed all forms of intimacy, to the tail end of the day when they are both exhausted and then wonder why they do not get the best out of their lovemaking.

The first thing to do when trying to improve conditions for sex is to set aside enough time so that you stand at least a fairly good chance of enjoying your lovemaking.

Choosing the best time of day can make a real difference too. Some people are at their sexiest in the mornings and others at night. If you both have different time clocks you can take it in turns so that you both enjoy the chance to have sex at a time which best suits you.

The time of the month can also make a difference for many women, and hence their men. Most women are at their sexiest just before or just after a period, or right in the middle of the cycle, so it makes sense to organize most sexual activity around these times. The best way to discover exactly what is the best time for sex is for the woman to chart her sexiness on a piece of paper for several months, recording how arousable she feels each day and how enjoyable her orgasms are when she has them. The couple can then organize

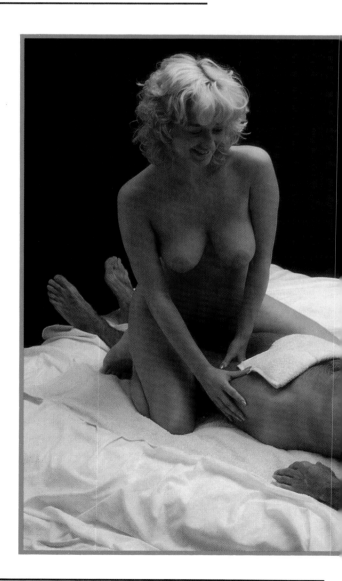

MAKE YOUR BEDROOM SEXIER

Although it is obviously possible to make love anywhere, most couples find that the best conditions can be obtained in their bedroom where they feel private and intimate. Your love nest should be reasonably soundproof, easily heated, have either candles or lighting that can be dimmed, have facilities for playing tapes or records, a lockable drawer or cupboard for sex toys and erotica, and anything else that particularly appeals.

A good bed is vital. One that is not too saggy makes things much better. A bed that sags does not support the woman's pelvic area and although this can, to some extent, be remedied by putting pillows under her bottom, this is often uncomfortable and even awkward. A bed should also ideally be as large as possible to allow you to indulge your creativity.

Keep some paper hankies handy near the bed so you can wipe yourselves afterwards. Have all your contraceptives, sex toys and whatever else you will need in a cupboard or drawer close at hand so that everything is easily accessible with the minimum of effort and disruption to the proceedings.

It is not difficult to lose the pleasure of the moment by having to put in your diaphragm though, of course, it could be put in by the man as part of foreplay.

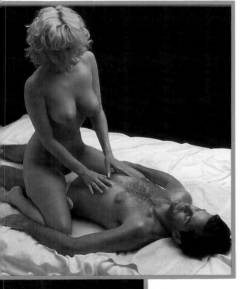

Sensual massage is one of the best ways to help you and your partner rid yourselves of the daily cares and allow you to be at your most relaxed. When massaging your partner, listen carefully to what he asks you to do and follow his instructions carefully

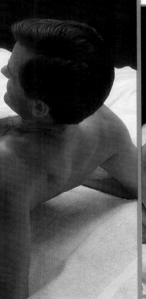

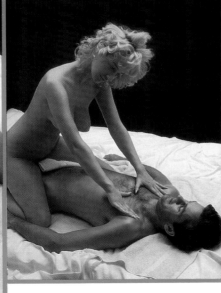

their sex life to take account of these natural rhythms.

Although quickie sex has its merits, most couples like to be able to spend some time together in loving and intimate behaviour as a prelude to intercourse itself. This means dedicating some time during which you will not be disturbed. This could call for some fairly drastic changes in the way you organize your life. If, for example, you are in the habit of watching TV until very late, this will almost certainly have to go.

Put aside an evening a week, which you keep totally free for yourselves, to do something sexy together. This will sometimes involve making love, on other occasions enjoying non-genital activities. Massaging one another, bathing together or cuddling while talking are all important ways of communicating intimately with your partner.

On a more ambitious level, you can try to make larger amounts of time for each other by taking a few days off together. This frees you to explore each other in a way that is rarely possible in the hurly-burly of daily life.

Get away from home and book into a hotel for a long weekend or, if you can, take a short holiday together. Breaks such as these can work wonders for your sex life as you re-learn about each other and increase the value you place on each other.

PERSONAL HYGIENE AND PREPARATION

Sex goes better if the couple have prepared their bodies beforehand. Lovemaking can be unpleasant because of poor hygiene and preparation.

Always have a bath if you are thinking of having sex. Make sure that your hair and teeth are clean and that your nails are clean and cut. A common complaint from women is that their man's fingers are stained with nicotine or his nails are too long or rough. None of these things make a woman too keen to have his fingers in, or even near, her vaginal area.

Wash your genitals carefully so that you smell pleasant. Many men neglect such matters and are less than scrupulously clean, and then complain that their partners are not keen on fellating them.

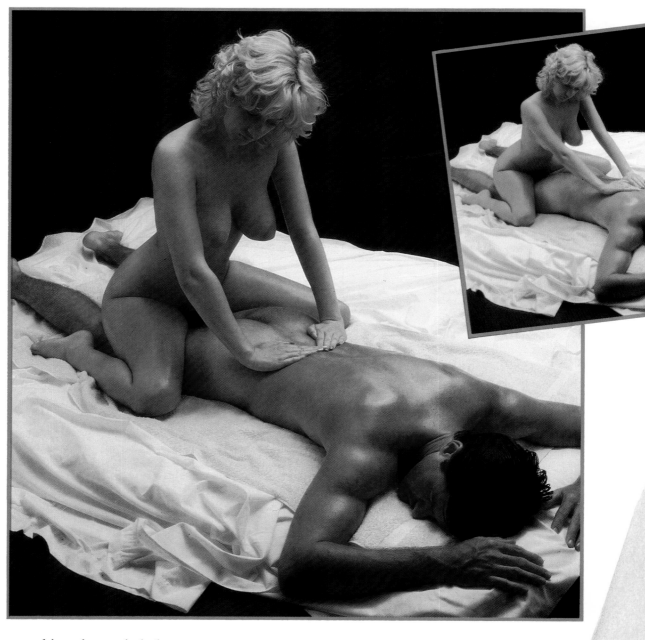

When washing the genitals be sure not to use a heavily-perfumed soap because this can mask the natural smells of the area which are put there by nature to turn on your partner. Similarly, when washing under your arms it is essential to remove stale sweat, but it is not necessary to use deodorant or once again you will mask the natural body odours.

BODY HAIR
People's views on body hair in both sexes differ enormously, but most men do little if anything to their body hair (except on their face) and most women remove hair from everywhere except around their genitals.

Men who have a heavy beard growth can be very stubbly by early evening and this can be a real turn-off

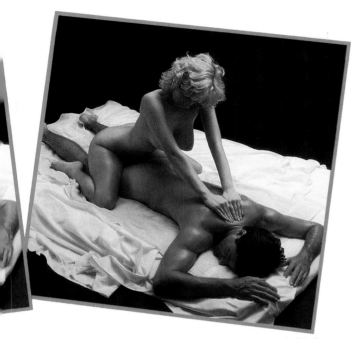

Once you have massaged his chest, stomach and thighs, turn him over and start on his back. You can either work your way up or down his torso, but be sure to pay special attention to the area at the back of the neck and across his shoulders. This region is particularly prone to tension and you may have to spend some time there

to those women who do not much like their face, or indeed anywhere else, being sandpapered by the stubble. The answer could involve shaving before making love, as well as in the morning, but if the prickly stubble offends your partner it is both worthwhile and considerate.

Most western men tend to like smooth-skinned women who have removed their body hair from all but the pubic area. Facial hairs are especially unacceptable to most couples, but tastes vary about how much of anything else should be removed. Stubbly legs are not much of a turn-on and some men dislike lots of pubic hair that creeps down the woman's thighs.

SEX AND MENSTRUATION
If the woman is menstruating, yet wants to make love in other ways than vaginally, she should ensure that she has changed her tampon recently and then washed her vulva.

Given this small amount of preparation she can now be kissed and sucked around her vulva. If she is in the heavier part of her cycle she can further ensure safety from leakage if she inserts a diaphragm before washing. This will hold back the flow for a couple of hours and then, when she has finished making love, she can use sanitary towels or a tampon as usual.

MAKE YOUR LIFE MORE EROTIC
Increasing the erotic level of our lives is one way to make us feel more in the mood for lovemaking. Sexy videos, girlie magazines, erotic books, sexy undies, sex toys and aids can all help to enhance the mood and make sex more likely to happen. Give one another little presents of sexy or romantic things so that every

Most women best know how to arouse themselves, so try to overcome any shyness you may have and let your partner watch you masturbate. This will allow him to see what you like best and in future lovemaking sessions he can incorporate what he learns into foreplay and increase the enjoyment for you both

two weeks or so you top up your fund of erotic goodwill between you.

MASTURBATE MORE
Unless you are already enjoying a very active sex life you will probably benefit from masturbating more frequently. Women particularly experience an increased

quality in their sex life once they start to masturbate more. Some women trying this approach to improving the conditions for sex find that they are thinking about sex much of the time and are thus ready and willing more often than they previously were.

Masturbating more frequently encourages the formation of new fantasies and, in women particularly, keeps the genitals in an almost permanently semi-aroused state. In men, more frequent masturbation means that they are less likely to be trigger happy and this can be of real value in the younger man.

For older men, this is not such a problem. Taking the pressure off with more masturbation may not be useful or necessary.

Learning to masturbate each other can increase your knowledge of what best turns on your partner, so this can be well worth trying if the conditions for sex are to be improved.

LEARN SENSUAL MASSAGE

Some couples enjoy sex less than they otherwise could, simply because they jumped too quickly for the hurly-burly of everyday life straight in to an intimate and sexual situation with little or no time in between to get used to each other. Sensual massage is a wonderful buffer between the two worlds.

The idea is that partners massage each other in turn in a way that is aimed solely at pleasing the one who is being massaged. This involves all kinds of feedback from the receiver to the giver – at least in the early days while the giver is learning what is best for his or her partner. Once a pattern of maximum

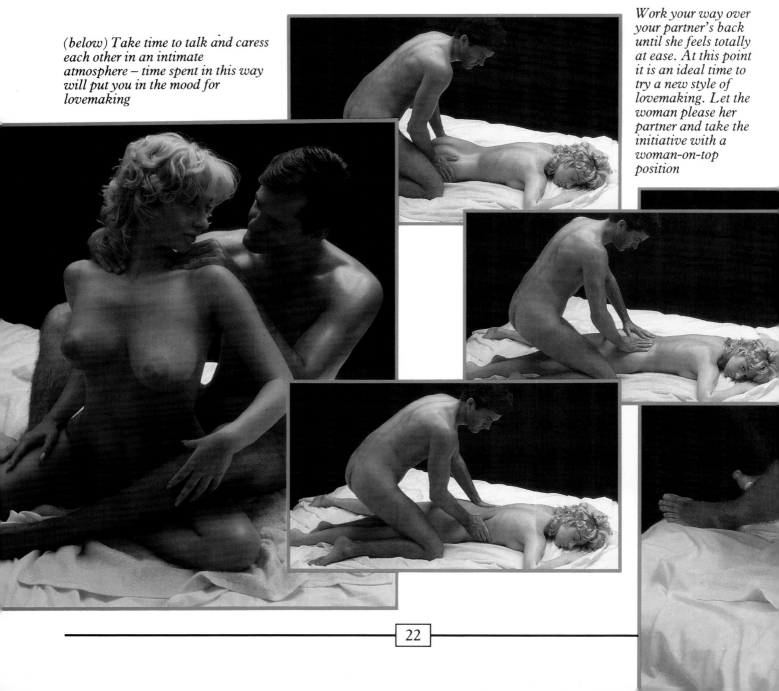

(below) Take time to talk and caress each other in an intimate atmosphere – time spent in this way will put you in the mood for lovemaking

Work your way over your partner's back until she feels totally at ease. At this point it is an ideal time to try a new style of lovemaking. Let the woman please her partner and take the initiative with a woman-on-top position

pleasure has been established, little or no verbal communication is necessary.

It all happens at the subconscious level, through grunts and moans of approval or tiny appreciative movements. However it occurs, a sensitive couple can, within a very few weeks, learn what best pleases each other during massage.

Sensual massage is not necessarily a prelude to lovemaking, although it might be on occasions. The most important thing is to ensure that it does not become a pleasure that is seen to be conditional upon sex following on. Make sensual massage an end in itself and not a stepping stone to sex and you will derive a lot more pleasure and relaxation out of it.

More to the point, it will set the conditions for intercourse at just the right level. The relaxation and trust that builds up during massage greatly helps both partners to become physically and mentally attuned to each other and ready for sex.

Apart from quickie sex, most people like to take time to unwind and to feel at ease being intimate. Sensual massage is perhaps the perfect way to do this and helps create very loving conditions for sex. It is an unselfish expression of caring for your partner.

Once the man is relaxed, he can then set about returning the compliment. Using a perfumed body oil will soften the woman's skin and the delicate scent will add to the atmosphere of the occasion

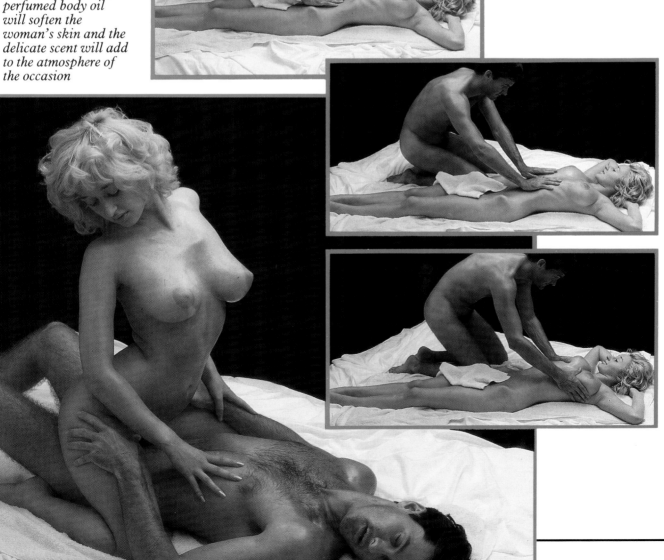

DRESSING FOR SEX

Clothes are an extension of love's visual vocabulary. And dressing sexily can be just as important to lovemaking as the undressing that follows

Dressing for sex is something most of us do subconsciously, but only rarely do we give it the thought and attention it truly deserves. This is a shame, because in the world that judges by appearances, clothes are love's visual vocabulary – learn to speak their language and your partner will sit up and listen. In turn, that means better, more exciting, and fulfilling sex — for both of you.

Clothing as a device for transmitting powerful sexual signals has long been recognized. History is full of sexy dressers. An 8th-century Chinese courtesan is credited with inventing the brassière, not as a means of supporting and uplifting her breasts, but of concealing them to entice and mystify her jaded lover.

Medieval Europe witnessed the growth of the codpiece – a garment that originated as a small patch for protecting the male genitals, but which by the 15th century had assumed such monstrously phallic proportions that its wearers became as incapacitated in the bedroom as their armour made them on the battlefield.

Even the prudish Victorians, renowned for fainting at the merest mention of a milky-white thigh, contrived to dress their men in tight breeches and their women in bosom-elevating, waisted waspies.

Nor is the idea of overtly sexual dress confined exclusively to advanced civilisations. The power of clothing to titillate and torment is universal and time honoured – a fact which prompted one 19th-century African chief to go as far as banning the wearing of them altogether in an effort to discourage licentious thoughts among his tribe.

DISPLAY, STIMULATION AND FANTASY

Drawing on many instances of men and women dressing, rather than undressing, for sex, theorists of the 20th century have pinpointed three key areas in which clothing fulfils an important sexual function.

First, we use clothes as 'plumage' to attract and excite a mate in much the same way as a male peacock displays its tail feathers. Attraction is mainly about body langage, and by adorning our body in appealing clothes we can make certain parts 'speak' more loudly.

Second, clothing can be sexually stimulating in a purely physical sense, perhaps because it mimics or even exaggerates the textures and sensations of the body that we associate with sexual caresses. There are clear parallels to be drawn between the supple, slightly damp feel of latex or rubber and the smooth pre-coital sweatiness of human skin. Less obviously, a fur coat can enhance these tactile qualities by virtue of its strongly contrasting colour and texture, as can a plain white shirt against a hairy chest.

But it is the third function of clothing – as a

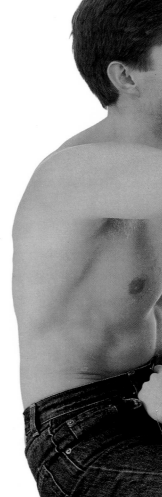

Our clothes may express a great deal about the kind of person we are, and enhance what we consider to be our best physical features

physical manifestation of sexual fantasy – that offers the most potential for experiment and eventual fulfilment. For, just as actors and actresses 'dress for the part' in order to make their characters more believable, so can the rest of us dress to give physical expression to that most erotic of human faculties – the imagination. And in an age when fashion is a multi-million-pound industry, and most of us can afford to splash out on our wardrobes occasionally, the scope for dressing sexily is wider than ever before.

DRESSING TO ATTRACT

When asked why they spend a fortune on clothes that have no apparent practical purpose, or spend many hours in front of the mirror adjusting a troublesome hem or tie, most people reply that they want 'to look good'. But what does looking good really mean? In almost every case it is a polite way of saying, 'I want to attract a mate'.

For the young, free and single, dressing to attract begins hesitantly – and sometimes painfully embarrassingly – with the onset of puberty. During this early exploratory phase, the idea is generally to copy friends, spurred on by the feeling that if you do not

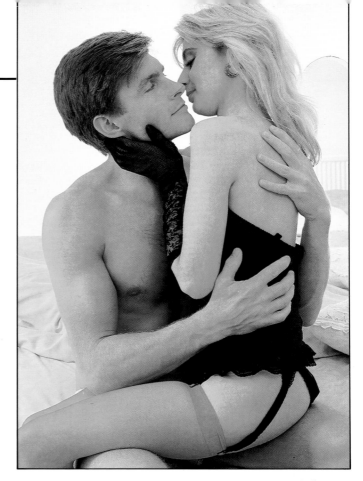

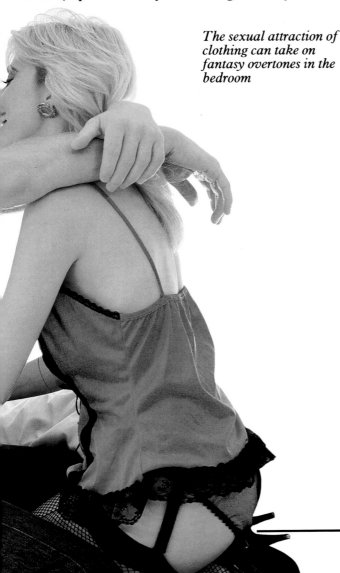

The sexual attraction of clothing can take on fantasy overtones in the bedroom

dress like they do you will subsequently be left out.

The shy 13-year-old who one day swaps her school uniform for a bra and blouse that emphasize her developing breasts is not automatically stating her desire to find a bedmate. She is simply expressing a wish to be found acceptable and 'attractive' by her friends.

It just so happens that these teenage definitions of 'attractiveness' are exactly those by which men will judge her in years to come. Nor does this desire to dress attractively in a socially acceptable sense disappear in adulthood. If you were to overhear work colleagues of your own sex commenting that you look 'a mess', the chances are you would be upset. This is because implicit in what they were saying would be the idea that you looked unattractive to members of the opposite sex – a condition that most of us instinctively try to overcome.

Dressing to attract is, therefore, a basic human need, but one which goes far beyond the desire simply to entice and entrap a mate. Even if you are happy and secure in a relationship, wearing clothes which attract the opposite sex is still a highly necessary occupation, if only because looking attractive makes you feel desirable.

All this not only works wonders for your self-respect, it also serves to act as a positive force in your lovemaking.

WHAT IS ATTRACTIVE DRESS?

Sexually attractive clothes are those which emphasize the parts of the body we find most attractive and disguise those we do not, the ultimate goal being to present to others an 'ideal' male or female form.

This 'ideal' form varies widely not only from culture to culture but from generation to generation, according to the dictates of fashion.

Consequently a Tonganese man would be probably no more likely to fall for a willowly model type than his European counterpart would for a plump Polynesian princess. (In Tonga, where fashion moves at a more leisurely pace than in London's Kings Road, the heavier a woman is, the more desirable she is considered.) Yet despite the variations, a look at the world-wide history of sexy dressing through the ages reveals a surprisingly universal pattern; one in which the same combinations reveal themselves again and again transcending time and culture.

In women, clothes which emphasize the breasts (especially the cleavage), narrow the waist and show off the shape of the hips and buttocks all make repeated appearances. So, too, do garments which offer a suggestion to a male observer of possible access to these important areas.

Legs are a consistent 'turn-on' feature. Dress performs both a revelatory role – for example, the mini skirt – and a shape-enhancing one – high heels, the pencil skirt or skin-tight jeans.

Among men, the accent is on clothes which make the shoulders and back appear broad, the neck and chest strong, and the hips and buttocks small and firm-muscled. Consider, for example, the almost continuous popularity in western society of short but padded jackets and tight, body-hugging trousers. Men, too, have contrived a form of dress which continues to emphasize the above characteristics while effectively disguising those less desirable by-products of middle age – sagging muscles and a pot belly. Now you know why the boss is so insistent that his male employees wear suits.

Moving from reality to fantasy, designer-label suits which imply wealth, style and – most importantly – power, can be just as great a 'turn-on' in the mind of the beholder as obviously sexy skin-tight jeans that reveal every bulge, or figure-hugging shirts slashed open to the waist.

EXPRESSING YOUR OWN SEXUALITY

How you put the theory of attractive dressing into practice depends as much on the kind of partner you wish to attract (or like the thought of attracting) as it does on how you see your own attractiveness. Dress like a prostitute or a nun and you will probably be treated like one.

But in between lies vast scope for you to express your own sexuality through what you wear. And during the course of finding out just where you stand on the sexy dressing scale, the following points are all

(below) Luxurious clothing is an automatic turn-on to almost any man

(right) Keep some clothes on during lovemaking for an entirely new erotic appeal

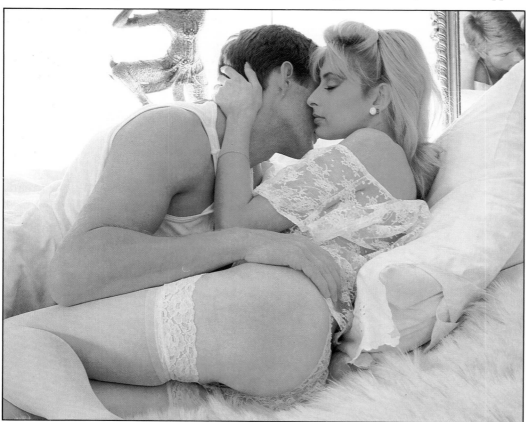

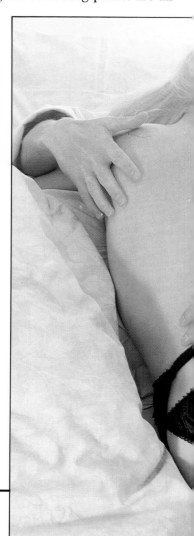

worth a great deal more than just a passing thought.

First, do not get bogged down or feel dictated to by fashion. Just because the well-rounded look may not be 'high fashion' does not mean to say that as a woman with a large bust you have to resort to shapeless smocks and armour-plated bras like your grandmother used to wear.

Make the most of your curves within the current limits of fashionable dress and let the admirers fight it out. Remember, there are just as many devotees of the fuller figure as there are admirers of girls who have a rather more boyish build.

Second, make the most of what your body has to offer and be realistic about the places that perhaps are not always quite what they once were or you would like them to be. As a woman, do not waste time squeezing a bottom that is a little on the large side into too-tight jeans when well-cut loose trousers could easily transform a problem rear into an asset. Likewise, as a man with a paunchy middle, you would be well advised to save the money you were going to spend on that T-shirt or figure-hugging sports shirt and invest it instead in the skills of a good tailor.

Third, think carefully about the sexual image you want to project and dress accordingly. A low-cut dress may be just what is required to get the boys on the building site worked up, but if your dream man is a sensitive, sophisticated type who appreciates women, you could find yourself attracting entirely the wrong people if you choose such an explicitly sexual outfit.

Above all, remember that dressing to attract is not about looking like a model or conforming to any set rules. It is about making the most of what you have got and wearing your clothes with style and grace rather than allowing fashion to dictate what you should wear – whether it suits you or not.

DRESSING FOR THE BEDROOM

If you can take the plunge and step out of your daily (or nightly) bedroom routine, the power of clothing to excite or enhance the lovemaking ritual can really begin to make itself apparent.

The same rules as 'dressing to attract' still apply, but in the bedroom there is a subtle shift from the role of clothing as attraction devices, to that of physical stimulant and aid to fantasy.

Dressing for the bedroom is much the same as presenting your partner with an elaborately wrapped Christmas gift. The content may be known, but how much more exciting to disguise it with layers of attractive adornment, casting doubt in the mind of the recipient as to the prize that awaits them at the end of their quest.

Sexual excitement is about anticipation – of the 'unseen', and imagined. Those high-necked, floor-length, pale cotton nighdresses that button down to the floor have never lost their appeal – and even the most uninterested lover should reach fever pitch (if that is the desired reaction) by the time he unbuttons it down to the knees.

EROTIC POTENTIAL
Clothes, in all their variety, present you with almost limitless opportunities to explore this powerfully erotic world.

Where dressing for the bedroom differs greatly from dressing to attract is that it is a more personal affair, and one in which your partner's preferences and tastes must necessarily take precedence over your own preconceptions about what constitutes sexy dressing.

This in turn means taking the time and trouble to find out – do not fall into the all-too-common trap of spending hours dressing in a slinky negligee, only to have it received with barely disguised amusement by a partner whose particular turn-on is a sporty nightshirt and a natural 'little-girl-lost' look.

Nor can you afford to let the whole world in on your secret. By all means dress like a prostitute or macho he-man, if that is what excites your partner – but not in public, or the chances are they will mistake your carefully prepared costume for a blatant attempt to attract another mate.

LOOK, LISTEN AND LEARN

To be a successful bedroom dresser you have to turn detective-cum-spy. Start by learning to spot those little clues by which everyone betrays their sexual desires. When your partner tells you that you look 'nice', make a note of what you are wearing and try find out more about exactly what prompted that particular response.

Have your mental note-pad handy when eyes pop out on stalks at the outfits of cinema or television stars. Try to pinpoint where the attraction lies and what part clothes play in the fantasy.

And, once you have completed your basic training, become more adventurous by turning conversations round to the subject of sexy dress. Magazines and videos can be particularly helpful here, by providing a starting point. Often you can learn plenty from a negative response – by exclaiming 'she looks sexy' and receiving a discouraging 'Oh no she doesn't' in reply, you at least know what your partner does not like, and soon you can piece together a mental picture of what they do like.

On no account adopt the bull-in-a-china-shop approach and come right out with, 'I want to dress sexily for you – what do you like?' By doing so you break the spell of unexpected fantasy upon which the real magic of sexy dress relies.

And once you have assembled enough information to put your plans into practice, bear in mind that dressing for the bedroom should start long before you pass through the boudoir door. Always remember that you are dealing with fantasy and the thrill of the unexpected – conditions that must be coaxed, teased and drawn out of your partner. As with lovemaking itself, build slowly towards a climax, offering oh-so-discreet hints as to what may be coming along the way.

DRESSING FOR HIM

As a woman, one of the following scenarios should at least give you some ideas on how to prepare yourself for sexy dressing.

Just before a dinner party or night out with friends, 'forget' to put on any knickers, and instead wear stockings and suspenders under a slinky dress that gives you the chance to let slip a tantalizing glimpse of thigh.

When the two of you are alone, mention casually

DRESSING TO UNDRESS

HER FOR HIM

☐ The age-old 'frilly underwear' combination of stockings, suspenders, lacy bras and exotic knickers is still a classic turn-on for many men. But you may well be able to make more of their sexual allure by being aware of variations and how they can be perceived:

White and frilly suggests an innocent, essentially feminine – and perhaps even submissive – role.

Black can be 'naughtier' or more 'sluttish' – or, if the quality is high, sophisticated and woman-of-the-worldish.

Skin-tight leather and latex with zip fastenings points to female domination, especially when teamed with lots of chains and spiky-heeled stilettos.

☐ The 'Sexy Schoolgirl' is another favourite, particularly when combined with adult underwear. The main rule is that clothes should be tight and revealing.

☐ The fresh-faced 'tomboy' look is becoming increasingly popular. Keep things natural – freshly-washed casually worn hair and no make-up are a must. Short, sporting nighties and oversized cotton nightshirts are the standard garb, while white stockings add a touch of unabashed naughtiness.

☐ The 'Professional Woman' look – strict, schoolmarm, tough businesswoman – is arousing to men because of the thrill suggested by seducing the untouchable. Wear severe suits and old-fashioned blouses over the naughtiest underwear you can find.

☐ The 'servant' look attracts the man who likes to dominate in the bedroom – nurses' and French maids' uniforms are classic examples.

☐ The 'French tart' look is sexy – even sluttish. Fishnet tights, basques, net T-shirts and slit skirts are all firm favourites, as are thigh-high 'kinky' boots and lace-up stilettos of the dominatrix.

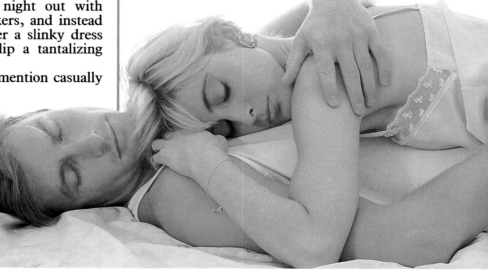

□ The 'femme fatale' look may borrow from any of the above, but in this case it must be tempered by immaculate dress sense and subtly sophisticated accessories. Underwear is naughty, but so too are necklines, backs and skirt slits – providing it's all done with the utmost good taste.

HIM FOR HER

The following stereotypes are all essentially pre-bedroom dressers, but if everything goes according to plain their styles should make their presence felt once the clothes are eventually peeled of.

□ The butch he-man. Leather jackets, tight denim jeans, white or checked shirts opened discreetly, white T-shirts – the classic masculine 'wild boy' look as exemplified by Marlon Brando in the film *On the Waterfront*.

□ The sportsman. Loose-fitting sports gear which somehow manages to show all the right bumps and bulges. Plus boxer shorts or swimming trunks for when things get hot.

□ The Latin lover. White tuxedo or expensive casual clothes in adventurously bright colours, trousers tight but well cut, shoes expensive.

□ The sensitive poet. Faded, tattered jeans and loose-fitting shirts – a deathly pallor is a must to complete the image.

□ The pop star. Unlimited potential here. Dress as far over the top as your imagination and budget will allow, but keep an ear open for what kind of music she is playing or you could get left behind.

□ The 'toff'. Dinner jacket, bow-tie, cummerbund – even a top-hat and cape won't go amiss. Everything should be classically tailored, made to measure and well pressed. Dress with an eye for detail.

how hot you are and how 'lucky' it is that you forgot a certain item of clothing. Later, in another private moment, find an excuse to step up the action by revealing a fleeting flash of suspender top, after which you can act as if nothing had happened.

Back at home, keep your cool and invite him to help you off with your dress. If, by this time, you still have not got a passionate raging bull on your hands, then you cannot have done your homework properly – or he has had too much to drink.

DRESSING FOR HER

As a man, dressing sexily for the bedroom often means beginning the evening by wearing your most flattering outfit – whether a smart suit or casual gear. But this in itself is not a guarantee of success later on.

Unless the personality matches up to the way you are dressed, the whole illusion may be shattered. And later, when, with luck, you reach the bedroom, do not let yourself down by undressing in a way that makes you look more like Coco the Clown.

Remember that, as far as she is concerned, you are playing a mild fantasy role that must be seen through to the end. The whole effect will be completely ruined if you have removed all your clothes except for your socks. Socks always come off before trousers unless you are aiming for a comic effect.

DRESSING SEXILY IS FUN

Once you have broken down the barriers between you and put to rest the myths that dressing sexily is 'stupid' or 'perverted', the most effective way to get the best of what clothes have to offer your sex lives is to invent 'games' in which you both have a fantasy role.

Switch off completely from the usual 'you', start acting, and you immediately banish the self-conscious-ness that often inhibits couples from expressing their desires through dress.

Before long you could easily find yourselves dressing as wildly as your fantasies will allow. And where the art of turning your partner on through what you wear is concerned, that is not a bad goal for a couple to work towards.

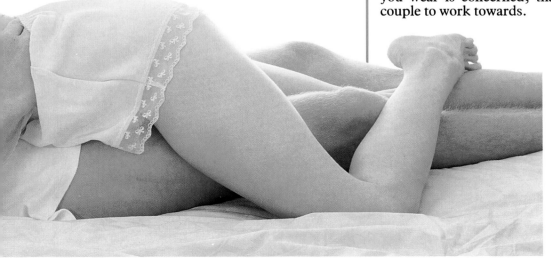

BREASTS AND SEX

A woman's breasts are her most obvious sexual characteristic; and, regardless of their shape and size, they can give pleasure and excitement to her and her lover

In the western world, women are probably more obsessed with their breasts than ever before, partly – if not entirely – because today's men are similarly obsessed. In a world in which women often have short hair and wear trousers, and are generally eroding men's traditional roles, men (and to a lesser extent women themselves) tend to see breasts as the one sexual difference they cannot hide, and so, if anything, emphasize their importance.

The media, and the 'girlie magazines' in particular, worship breasts in a totally unnatural way which makes many women feel insecure and men dissatisfied. Clever photography and posing can do wonders for a modestly-endowed woman, but the reader sees only the finished shot and the woman reader may wonder why she cannot look like the pneumatic beauties her partner so admires.

BIG-BREASTED WOMEN

Admiration for the big-breasted women stems in part from the Hollywood era of film stars with hourglass-shaped figures. Since the 1940s, boys have grown up with the idea that big breasts are sexy. Not only are big-breasted women thought to be intrinsically more interested in sex, but their very appearance is traditionally thought to carry more sex appeal to men. The combination of looks, plus the fact that the men believe such women are more interested in sex, conspire to attract men to women with big breasts.

Of course, it might be true to say that some women who grow up with relatively big breasts are more interested in sex than are their smaller-breasted

Whether gently kissed, squeezed or nibbled, a woman's breasts, no matter what size, can give her exquisite pleasure. The wise lover devotes much time to his partner's breasts

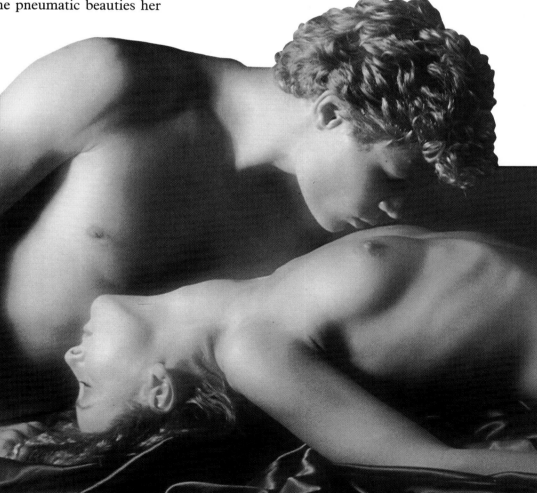

sisters. From adolescence onwards they will have been unable to ignore the interest their shape arouses in men and, indeed, in other women, and they cannot help but be aware that big breasts are considered sexy.

ONLY PART OF SEX APPEAL

The danger for big-breasted women comes when they start believing that their sex appeal starts and ends with their breasts. It is a very superficial relationship which is based only on each partner's tacit acceptance of the beauty of a part of one of their bodies.

Women with beautiful faces have often found themselves in a similar situation and, even worse, have found – like several film stars – that their whole value amounts to little more than a pretty face.

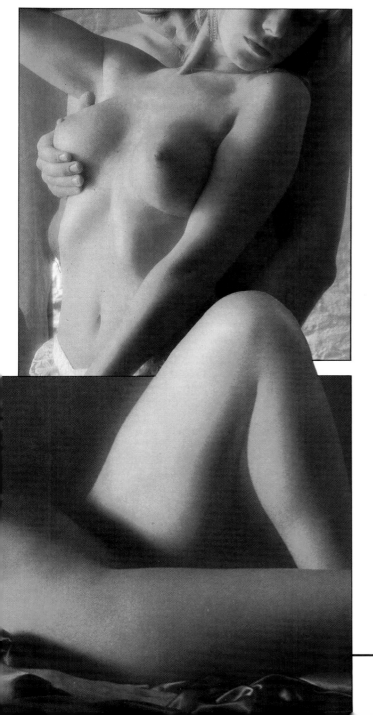

THE IDEAL BREAST?

Most men and women understand that small-breasted women can be just as sexy, and can have just as much sex appeal, as big-breasted ones. This is not to say, though, that individual preferences as to the look of breasts should not exist. It is difficult to wipe out a person's culturally-inherited values of physical beauty. Different people have always had their own ideas of what constitutes ideal female physical beauty, and many of these ideals have differed enormously from those western society holds today.

And it seems that society's ideal breast image is showly changing anyway. The ideal woman, is portrayed by the media, is neither very slim, nor very curvy. She is neither particularly big- or small-breasted. This perhaps reflects the enormous variety of fashion, hairstyles, makeup, popular music and drama available today, which are incompatible with the concept of a stereotyped woman.

OTHER INFLUENCES

Fashions, advertising and male conditioning all contrive to make women increasingly breast-conscious, and although many women do not see their breasts as being of especial sexual significance compared with the rest of their bodies, many are virtually forced to do so by pressure from outside. This leads some women to see the role of their breasts as exclusively sexual, never considering any other role for them.

This means that when anything goes wrong (they find a lump, for example) they are terrified to go to a doctor just in case it means that their main sexual symbol will have to be removed, On average, a woman with a lump in her breast waits for six months before seeking medical help. This delay would not occur if the lump were on her foot or another less sexually important part of her anatomy.

VULNERABILITY

The media and advertising can have a potent and lasting effect on a young girl as she grows up, but there are other influences. Girls compare their breast development with each other and with their mother's, both in reality and in fantasy, and for most girls their breasts are the first manifestation of their awakening sexuality. They can be intensely proud of them and, quite naturally, want to display them to their best advantage.

At first, this produces an ambivalent attitude and a sense of guilt as men (and particularly their fathers) begin to notice that they are not little girls any more, but young women. Indeed, many adolescent girls hide their budding breasts from their fathers because of this new-found awareness.

SELF-EXPLORATION

As a young girl's breasts develop, she experiments with handling them and soon finds that it feels good. Some girls go through a phase of allowing other girls to play with their breasts and this is completely normal.

(right) Begin breastplay gently – brushing the palm of your hand over the skin of her breasts, before approaching her nipples

(middle) Cupping a breast in your hand, use your mouth to kiss and caress the senstitive areola around the nipple itself

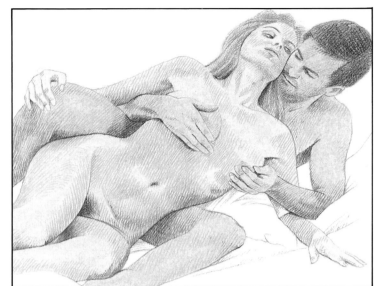
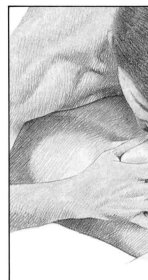

(right) Use your breasts to trace a tantalizing path up and down the length of his body, while he lies passive beneath you

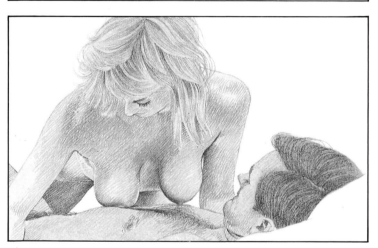
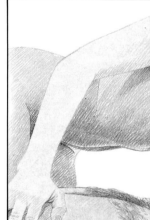

Many of us go through a homosexual stage during our sexual development but this is usually a prelude to heterosexual relationships. Once heterosexual contact starts, a girl realizes that boys like her breasts and so makes the most of it. At this stage the breasts become important sexual symbols and she starts to buy bras and to wear clothes that accentuate what Nature has given her.

BREASTS AND AROUSAL

During the earliest phase of sexual arousal, the first sign that anything is happening is that the nipples become erect. This comes about as the tiny, smooth muscles in them contract. One nipple often becomes erect before the other and erection can occur even without physical stimulation – in extremes of wind or temperature, for example.

Touching, by the woman herself or by her partner, usually hastens erection but it is not essential. The nipples increase in length and diameter as the woman becomes more excited and blood collects in and around them. This mechanism is rather like that which causes a penis to become erect.

SIZE AND SENSITIVITY
The size of the breasts and nipples has no bearing on how responsive they are sexually. Some women have exquisitely sensitive nipples which, when stimulated, bring them to orgasm within seconds, while other women's nipples are almost totally unresponsive. (Much the same is true of men.)

Nipple length during sexual arousal may increase by up to one centimetre and nipple width by up to half a centimetre. Average-sized nipples increase proportionately more than do larger ones. Generally, mouth stimulation (sucking and gentle licking) produces faster nipple erection than does stimulation with the fingers, but obviously this varies from woman to woman, and according to time and mood.

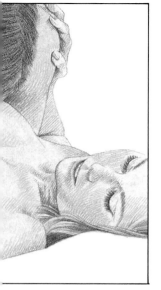
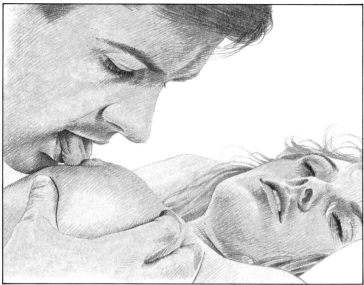

(left) With your tongue, lick and flick her erect nipple, then draw it into your mouth as her pleasure intensifies towards orgasm

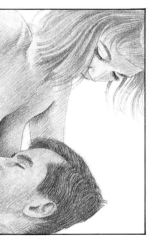
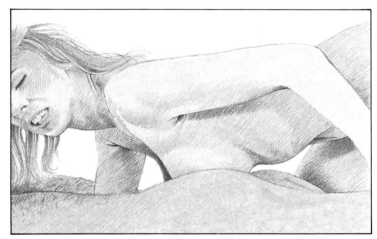

(middle) Now move your body up towards his face, caressing his chest with your hand, as your breasts brush against his mouth and eyes

(left) Then turn him over, and trace another path, this time travelling down his spine to the sensitive area between his buttocks

THE EXCITEMENT PHASE

Once the nipples are erect, the pattern of veins on the breasts can frequently become more marked and breasts begin to swell – sometimes by as much as 30 per cent of their usual volume. This swelling is most obvious in women who have not breastfed. Later on during this excitement phase, the areolae swell and, in light-skinned women in particular, the breasts may become covered with a faint red flush or measles-like rash which can also extend to cover the abdomen and neck. Some women, however, do not have a sex flush at all, and in others it appears very late.

THE PLATEAU PHASE

The next stage of sexual arousal is commonly known as the plateau phase. During this, the breasts swell to an even greater extent and the areolae especially become swollen. This swelling may be so marked that it makes the nipples appear shorter. In fact, the nipples are usually still swelling at this stage but are masked by the swelling of the areolae which increase even more dramatically at this stage.

ORGASM

At orgasm itself, women experience all kinds of sensations, of which some are related to their breasts. Some women like their breasts or nipples held very hard or even squeezed as they have an orgasm but, because the intensity of the other changes in the body is so great, it is easy for a man to damage his partner's breasts or nipples as she comes because she is much less sensitive to pain.

It makes sense to draw a line between what a couple finds pleasant and stimulating and what seems to produce damage. This is particularly true of biting the breasts or nipples during intercourse, so care is called for.

RESOLUTION

Once orgasm is over, the areolae return to normal. This marks the onset of the final phase of the sexual arousal cycle – the resolution phase. This change in the areolae gives the impression that the nipples are becoming erect again, but this is not so. They are simply more visible as the surrounding areas subside.

This increased prominence of the nipples is a good sign that the woman has had an orgasm. The sex flush begins to fade away and the breasts return to their former unexcited size.

At this stage many woman do not want their breasts touched because they are tender or so pleasantly 'satisfied' that further stimulation is positively unpleasant. Unlike men, though, many women are capable of several orgasms in succession and soon the breasts are ready for a new excitement phase.

BREASTPLAY

Almost all women say that they like their breasts to play some part in their lovemaking, so it is sad that so often men do not do to their women's breasts what they would most like to have done.

Many women complain that men are too rough (especially squeezing their breasts too much). They also find their partner places too much emphasis on breastplay too early in sexual arousal.

Another complaint – as so often in any sexual activity, common to both sexes – is that the man fails to ask what the woman herself wants. Many women play with their breasts and nipples when they masturbate, and could easily tell their men what they most like, if only they were asked.

WHAT WOMEN WANT
Provided a couple can talk to each other about their sexual preferences, it is up to the woman to tell her partner what she most likes and to school him in caressing her breasts in the way that suits her best.

Generally, most women want their breasts to be played with late in foreplay, rather than early on, and then very lovingly and gently. The only time a woman may want any roughness – if indeed she wants any at all – is very late when she is highly excited, as she approaches, or is having, an orgasm.

FOR HER

There are a number of things a man can do to his partner's breasts to increase her pleasure – both in foreplay and during intercourse.

☐ **Watch her as she masturbates** Take note on how she plays with her breasts and at what stage. Does the pressure increase as she approaches orgasm? What seems to stimulate her most?

☐ **Be gentle** Use the palm of your hand to brush lightly over her breasts. There are also a number of oils available – although baby oil is as good as any – that can be gently massaged into them. Go slowly around each breast, leaving the nipples until last.

☐ **Be guided by what she likes** Her nipples may become so sensitive that direct stimulation is painful.

☐ **Be imaginative** Use other parts of your body to tease and excite her. Flutter your eyelashes over her breasts, or use feathers or a piece of velvet, but be careful not to tickle. The line dividing arousal and tickling is a fine one.

☐ **Use your mouth together with your hands** Caress her elsewhere on her body or caress the other breast as well. Go round and round the nipple with your tongue, gently sucking and nibbling. As an added variation you can try using food or wine and eating or drinking them off her breasts. This will not only make them taste nice, but there is also something intensely erotic for a great many women in having their breasts bathed in food or liquid – particularly those with a

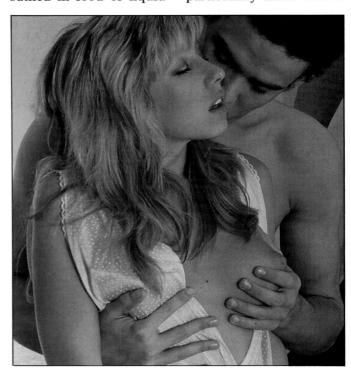

creamy texture – which their man hungrily laps up.

☐ **Use your penis** Tease and excite her by touching her with your penis, but do not ejaculate unless that is what she wants you to do. Use it instead to trace a path around each breast.

FOR HIM

There are few bigger turn-ons for a man than when his partner uses her body to tease and excite him. For the woman, this can be both exciting and flattering as she finds that she can use her breasts to bring her partner to a pitch of arousal – perhaps even to orgasm.

USING HER BREASTS TO TEASE
The breasts can be used on their own, or in conjunction with the rest of a woman's body, to arouse

her partner just about anywhere. Here the woman can assume an active role and allow the man to lie back and enjoy what she is doing to him.

☐ **Trace a path with one, or both, of your breasts** Cover the whole length of his body, avoiding only his genitals at this stage. Use your nipples to trace a light fluttering path and alternate this with pressing your breasts flat against his body.

☐ **Turn him over** Do the same over his back, using your nipples to trace a path over and between his buttocks.

☐ **Tease his breasts with yours** Some men have extremely sensitive nipples; others do not. If your man does, try putting some saliva – his or your own – on your breasts and rub them against his nipples. If you do not want him to touch you yet, use your hands to press down on his shoulders to restrain him.

☐ **Dangle your breasts over his erect penis** Use your nipples to trace a path up and down it.

☐ **Place his erect penis between your breasts** Ask him to hold them together or hold them together yourself and wrap them around the shaft of his penis. If he uses his hands, you can use your own to bring him to orgasm as you move your body rhythmically up and down. Intercourse between the breasts can be good in other positions as well – head to tail, the man sitting or on top, or with the woman kneeling. Experiment to find the position that suits you both.

Now you can allow him to take more active role. Lying beneath him, let him place his erect penis between your breasts, while you squeeze them together so that they envelop him like a vagina. Move your bodies together to bring him to the brink of orgasm

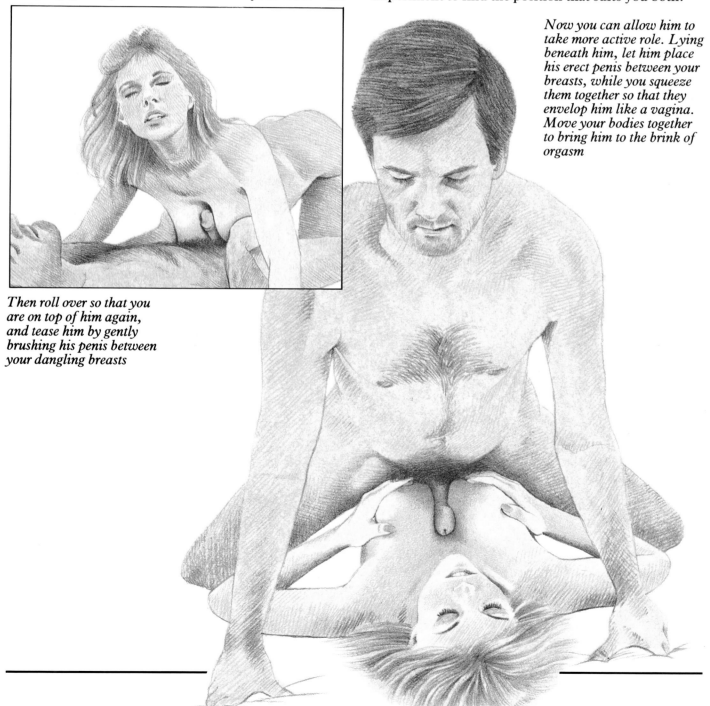

Then roll over so that you are on top of him again, and tease him by gently brushing his penis between your dangling breasts

FEMALE FANTASIES

In childhood, through adolescence to womanhood, females fantasize – and sexual fantasy becomes an important part of most women's sex lives

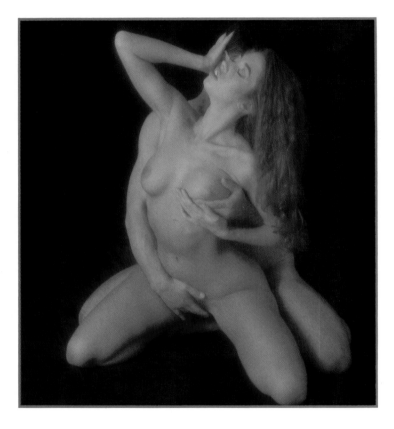

Many women inhabit a rich and varied world of sexual fantasy. A couple's sex life can be enriched and improved when such dreams are brought into play in lovemaking

Almost everyone fantasizes about sexual matters, but many claim not to do so. This paradox can be explained quite easily when the working of the unconscious mind is taken into account. Most of us in the western world are brought up with at least some negative notions about sex. We mostly think it is naughty, guilt-ridden or, in some other way, unacceptable – especially outside marriage. This means that for some, at least, fantasy material that surfaces during daydreaming or masturbation is immediately pushed back into the unconscious mind from whence it came for fear of having to confront it in the conscious mind. So it is that therapists seeing individuals who have unconscious fantasies can often unlock this barrier and 'allow' previously forbidden fantasy material to surface and so be enjoyed.

Sexually uninhibited people have no problem with fantasizing and their bank of fantasy material is large and ever-changing. Most of us have favourite fantasies that work well and for many they work as a kind of sexual talisman – they seem to bring luck and good fortune to the sexual encounter almost as if by magic.

HIDDEN FEMALE FANTASIES

Both sexes fantasize, but until recently it has been thought that women did so less than men. We all know about men's fantasies – they talk about them in locker rooms, around bars, in the form of dirty stories and so on – but women's fantasies have historically been kept in the dark. This is hardly surprising given that female sexuality is much more repressed than men's.

Part of the reason for this suppression has

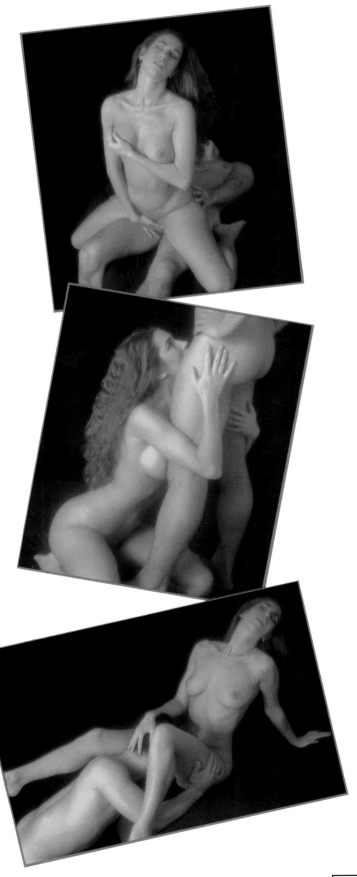

undoubtedly been the fact that many men, insecure as they are about their sexual performance and emotions, have tended to denigrate women's fantasies as being substitutes for the 'real thing' as if only frustrated women had fantasies and 'real women' were being totally satisfied by their men.

This is, of course, complete nonsense. Women have always been encouraged to be much more secretive about anything sexual. This has led, at least until very recently, to a sort of underground of sexual feelings and fantasies and, like all underground movements, gains power and strength from its very secrecy.

That most women fantasize sexually can now be in little doubt and with the current movement towards a more open expression of female sexuality, a lot more research is being done into the subject. A milestone in this movement was Nancy Friday's book *My Secret Garden*, which gathered together hundreds of fantasies from ordinary women who were prepared to share them. This book took the lid off the subject in a major way and made many men think seriously about the subject for the first time.

Even now, some years later, many men still find it difficult to think of their women fantasizing and, even if they can accept that they do, they cannot see why it should be necessary, especially if they are enjoying an active sex life. Clinical experience seems to show that, on the contrary, those women who have the best sex lives also have the richest fantasy lives.

WHAT DO WOMEN FANTASIZE ABOUT?

Women tend to fantasize about anything and everything and their sexual fantasies are very rich in content. What women say they fantasize about most is their current partner. Next in line is someone else they know, followed by a celebrity, strangers, animals and then other things. Some women, of course, have other fantasies, incestuous ones for example, that do not come to consciousness and these by definition cannot be recorded in the studies that have been done.

It is, of course, possible that women mislead researchers who ask about fantasies by tending to give the answers they think the questioner wants to hear, could best cope with, or which shows them in the best light. Thus fantasies about their partner seem acceptable and are those most readily volunteered. It could well be that this is not the true situation.

The other problem when trying to ascertain what women fantasize about is that the age, social class and sexual experience of the women being questioned will tend to influence the responses obtained. Studies of Californian undergraduates would, therefore, tend to produce rather different results from those of Scottish housewives, for example. But in spite of these problems, certain things do seem to occur.

☐ **Re-living a precious sexual experience** is almost certainly the most common of all female fantasies. This is used to conjure up the magic of a past occasion when everything seemed to go well. The content need not necessarily be all that sexual or genital. Many women's favourite fantasy of this kind involves a great deal of scene-setting (especially erotic places), mood memory and romantic thoughts. Most usually this type of fantasy involves the woman's current partner, but it may involve a past one.

☐ **Being overpowered physically** or even being 'raped' is the next most common fantasy in many surveys. Given that many women in our culture are so inhibited about sex, some need to be able to absolve themselves from the guilt associated with wanting sex and so create scenarios in which they have no responsibility for what happens – they are overwhelmed and thus have no say in the matter. This frees them, unconsciously, to enjoy the fantasy encounter whole-heartedly and without guilt.

☐ **Sex with more than one partner** features fairly commonly too. This fulfils, in fantasy, the need some women have to prove to themselves that they are desirable and fancied wildly by men in general, not just by their partner.

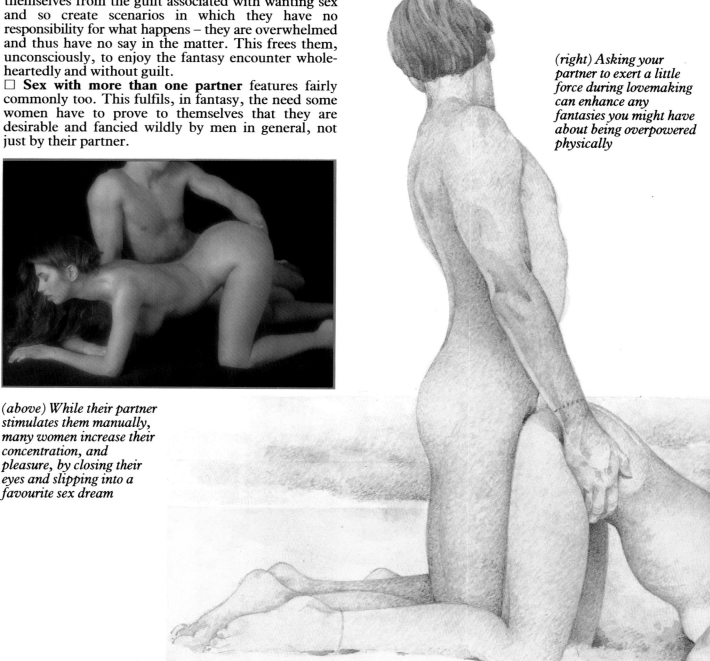

(above) While their partner stimulates them manually, many women increase their concentration, and pleasure, by closing their eyes and slipping into a favourite sex dream

☐ **Making love with a celebrity** is a type of fantasy that has almost become a stand-up joke. Many women feel easier about such fantasies because they are 'safe'. They are extremely unlikely to come true and, as such, the women can indulge in all kinds of wishful thinking that does not take the celebrity's needs or personal tastes into account.

So it is that a woman who would never be able in real life to gain the attention, let alone the bed, of such

(right) Asking your partner to exert a little force during lovemaking can enhance any fantasies you might have about being overpowered physically

a person can enjoy the fantasy nevertheless. This in turn enhances her own sexual ego and makes her more aroused for her non-celebrity lover.

☐ **Same-sex fantasies** are not at all unusual. Women who have this kind of fantasy are usually not homosexual but are turned on by the thought of sex with another woman. There are many causes for such fantasies, one of which is a disenchantment with men in general, or with their man in particular. A woman who feels this way retreats to same-sex fantasies to give herself a rest from the 'troublesome world of men'. Of course, some women are homosexual and will tend to fantasize about women on most occasions.

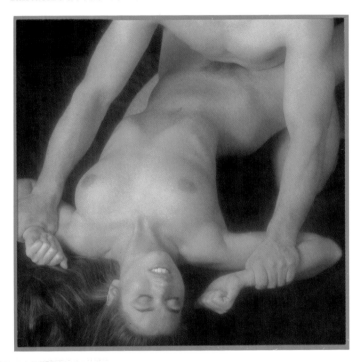

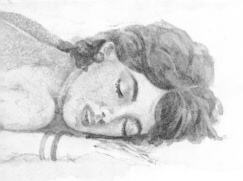

Using fantasy as a vehicle, many women transport their lovemaking from the bedroom to a romantic location and heighten their state of arousal in the process

FANTASY EXPLAINED

Why the sexual fantasies of women are so rich is a complex question and one open to debate. First, there is the 'underground' nature of these secret fantasies and the fact that they have grown as a result of their suppression by society. Next, many women are highly creative and have very fertile minds, especially on romantic and sexual matters. Women can experience many more physical pleasures in the sexual arena than men can and their rich fantasy life is just another part of this large sexual capacity. Most men are physically arousable only genitally and can only have one orgasm, unless they are very young. Most women have many erogenous zones and can be aroused by a whole host of different activities, both mental and physical. They can also have many orgasms in quick succession. All of this is mirrored in the average woman's fantasy life and some make use of their considerable bank of fantasies on most days of their lives.

WHEN DO WOMEN FANTASIZE
Although many women, just like men, fantasize in a day-dreaming sort of way when waiting in the supermarket queue or when on a bus, the vast majority of true sexual fantasies occur when masturbating. Few of us, of either sex, can become physically aroused at the drop of a hat – we need some sort of mental preparation. Fantasy primes the pump very effectively. According to one survey, 65 per cent of women use fantasy to create the mood when masturbating and it is possible that this is an underestimate. Clinical experience suggests that the vast majority of women use some sort of fantasy to get things going when they masturbate.

FANTASY AND FOREPLAY
The next most common time for fantasy to be used is during foreplay. Many women who do not feel like having sex at the time their partner wants it will draw on their fantasy pool to help get in the mood. This also happens, of course, when they do want sex. Either way, many women can progress fairly quickly from 'cold' to being highly aroused by using a favourite fantasy. About half of all women claim to use fantasy in this way.

FANTASY AND ORGASM
Some women only bring fantasy into play as intercourse progresses to its climax. They use it as a way of tipping themselves over the top into an orgasm – until this point they are in touch with their partner and the surroundings they find themselves in. For many women, however well a particular sexual encounter goes, and however much they love their man, climax eludes them for one of many reasons unless they can enhance the quality of their sexual arousal by using their highly personal fantasy.

Lastly, some women use fantasy only in particular

sexual situations such as when performing oral sex. To such a woman the reality of the situation may only become acceptable if they fantasize about someone or something else.

The vast majority of women then use fantasy to increase their level of sexual excitement although about a quarter say that they use it only to get things going. A small minority actually use fantasy to make them feel less sexy.

For some women, the intensity of their orgasms can be increased greatly if they leave reality behind and lose themselves in a world of fantasy when making love

average man does, but once they have got there, they can have more orgasms and remain in a state of arousal for longer than their partner.

Many men simply do not spend enough time arousing their women in the way they best like, or indeed need, so their partner finds herself making up the deficit in fantasy. Even those men who are excellent lovers must accept that, for some women, their drive for increased excitement leads them to fantasize to enhance things still further. It has been said in jest, but nonetheless has more than a grain of truth in it, that some women are 'greedy' in this way . . . and who can blame them?

MEN, WOMEN AND FANTASY

Women's fantasies can give rise to complications. Many, if not most, men find the whole notion of women fantasizing during sex threatening and even disgusting. Their shock is understandable but is ill-placed because several studies have found that well over half of all women fantasize when making love and clinical experience suggests that this figure is far lower than the reality of the issue.

Men who feel this way say that their women should be thinking only of them and should be keeping their mind on the job in hand, not thinking about their next door neighbour or Mel Gibson. Many men are truly upset by this and make a considerable fuss when they learn what is going on. They immediately interpret the woman's need to have such fantasies as being critical of their abilities to arouse her and make things happen to her. This is understandable given men's sexual insecurity, but is hardly excusable. What these men have to understand is that many women need a great deal more stimulation to become aroused than the

SEXUAL DAYDREAMING

For a few women who are very interested in sex, low-level sexual fantasies are an almost hour-by-hour part of their lives. These women find themselves thinking about sex in a sort of daydreamy way much of the time. Some of them do so because they are heavily involved in a sexy one-to-one relationship and others because they are not, but would like to be.

There is little doubt that the current vogue for romantic fiction – it is the most buoyant area in the whole of the publishing industry – reflects the needs some women have for fantasy on a daily, or even hourly, basis. Some women read several of these books a week, every week, and are aroused both sexually and romantically by them.

For many inhibited women to whom overt sexual activity is either unavailable, distasteful or thought to be sinful or naughty, such books are a lifeline because they 'allow' their sexual interests to be expressed under the guise of romance. In fact, the very inexplicit nature of most such books is the reason for their success. The reader can insert her own personal fantasies rather than have the author foist theirs upon her.

That romantic fiction is highly arousing to women, or at least to some of them, has been proven in laboratory experiments which measured very accurately women's sexual arousal before and after such material. It was found that women were just as aroused by these stories as were men by girlie magazines.

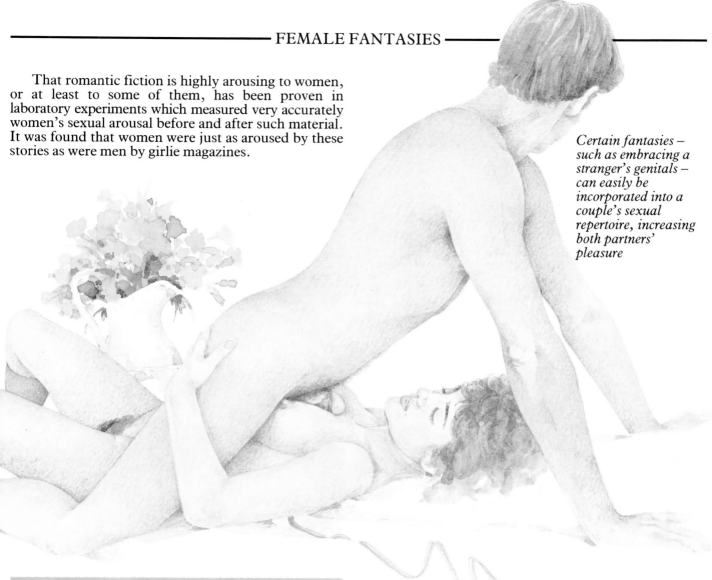

Certain fantasies – such as embracing a stranger's genitals – can easily be incorporated into a couple's sexual repertoire, increasing both partners' pleasure

COMPLICATIONS

On the vast majority of occasions, and for most women, fantasies are perfectly harmless and add greatly to the pleasure of the occasion. However, there can be problems, if only rarely.

Perhaps the most common problem, or potential problem, is when a woman finds that she is so hooked on a fantasy that she cannot have intercourse, or climax during masturbation without it. This may not, of course, greatly matter during masturbation but it often suggests that something is wrong with the woman's one-to-one relationship if she needs to distance herself from her man in this way during intercourse. Such a woman often finds that she does not want her man to talk, or in any way to intrude on her fantasy. This can be a real nuisance to the man because he realizes that she is miles away in another world and that he is simply the penis and the body that acts out the physical side of the act they are both involved in. This can destroy his pleasure totally. The wise woman does everything she can to make things less obvious.

Another drawback to using the same fantasy on a regular basis is that it can become a sort of conditioned reflex without which sex is impossible or joyless – not greatly different to a fetish. This is not all that harmful but means that the woman finds herself in a rut and that should anything happen to harm the fantasy she cannot function well or even at all. It pays to have a small bank of fantasies that can be called on at various times according to the mood.

OTHERS' FANTASIES

A good way of building up such a bank is to talk with other women, if you feel you can, or to read books about the fantasies of others. This usually opens doors that were previously totally closed.

Lastly, most fantasies are intensely personal but can be shared with a partner. There are however, dangers to doing so and caution must be the watchword. There is no limit to a fantasy's content, while it remains held within.

MALE
FANTASIES

At the onset of puberty, young boys add sexual fantasy to their development. As they grow into young men, their store of fantasies increases to include a wide range of images

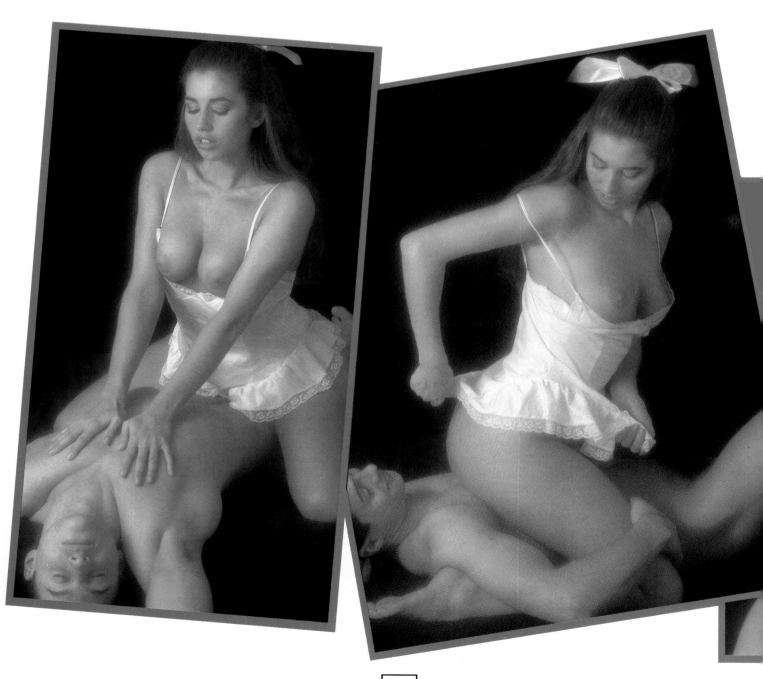

The main difference between male and female sexual fantasies is that men are much more likely to admit to them. This comes about because in western culture, males are more open about their sexuality and are, as a result, much less inhibited about admitting to the realities of it both to themselves and to others.

Little boys, just like little girls, fantasize about all kinds of non-sexual things and, as puberty beckons, they start to add sexual fantasy to their development. In the early teenage years, especially as boys begin to practise masturbation, possibly in the presence of other boys, they build fantasy into their sex lives from many sources.

A LEARNING PROCESS

As puberty approaches, males have a lot to learn when it comes to the practicalities of sex and it is at this stage that many start to take their learning very seriously indeed. Most boys of this age become highly interested in girls and, given that so much about the female body

For many men, exotic or 'naughty' underwear will be part of their favourite fantasies and, therefore, play an important part in their sex lives

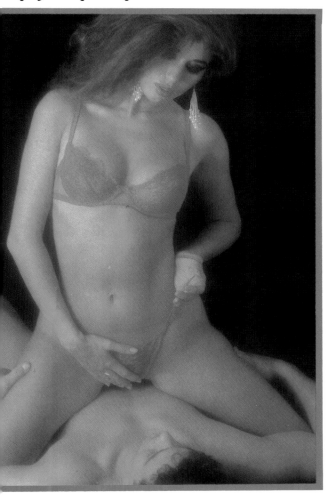

is hidden from view, they start to look at naked women in girlie magazines. In this way, they come to build up a picture of what women are really like and it is these early images that form the mental material for their masturbation fantasies.

PERSISTENT IMAGES

During puberty then, the average boy starts to put together his own personal bank of fantasies that work well for him. No one will ever know why it is that a particular image works at the time, but there is little doubt that far earlier childhood memories – albeit unconscious ones – play a vital part. Perhaps it was something he became aware of when he was as young as three or four – something his mother wore some years before – or perhaps he saw a neighbour or friend of his parents naked by mistake when changing for swimming. The possibilities are endless. Whatever the trigger was, he now favours certain images and rejects others, and all of this goes on quite unconsciously.

So, by the time that boys start to go out with girls seriously, they have many fantasies that they can call on to help arouse or even slow them down in a real-life sexual encounter.

PRIVATE FANTASIES

Men's fantasies have always been more openly expressed than those of women. Men talk more about sex than women do and locker room chat, bar room talk and men's magazines are awash with men's sexual fantasies.

Yet, most men are somewhat private about their own sex lives and often keep their personal fantasy material to themselves. The bonhomie around the bar is often only skin deep and, ironically, many men are more reluctant, in sexual and marital therapy, to talk about their fantasies than are women.

For some, the fantasy seems to have a kind of lucky charm effect and some men undoubtedly feel that to part with it to another could reduce its effect in the sexual situation. Men also tend to be very competitive. Perhaps some believe, however unconsciously, that to share their deepest fantasies in this way could open them up to unfair competition from another man, who might then use the knowledge to their sexual disadvantage.

WHAT DO MEN FANTASIZE ABOUT?

Although a common theme in women's fantasies is being overwhelmed by a strong man and being 'forced' to do sexy things 'against their will', very few men have fantasies of overpowering women. On the contrary, the women are usually compliant and willing, in response to his own fantasized power.

Even in the most detailed of sado-masochistic fantasies, most men do not usually receive any pleasure out of inflicting pain on the women but rather on forcing her to do something that transports her into new realms of delight and which she would not otherwise enjoy unless she was 'forced'.

In a sense, this is both selfless and totally self-centred. It is selfless because in the fantasy many men will go to enormous lengths to satisfy their women – often even being heroically selfless about it and putting their sexual needs last.

Yet, it is also selfish in that it bolsters the man's ego, proving to him that his woman, or at least the fantasy woman, finds him irresistible and the holder of the key to even greater sexual bliss.

These two need not, of course, be mutually exclusive, either in fantasy or real life. The man who feels good about arousing his partner to sexual delights she probably would not aspire to herself, takes nothing away from her. On the contrary, it is in the woman's best interests to encourage him to feel good about it.

MORE CREATIVE FANTASIES

Although women have a wide range of sexual fantasies, they fall into a few broad categories that cover the majority of women. This is less so for men. Men, as the sexual 'doers' in our culture, are perhaps more called upon to be more creative even in their most personal fantasy life. It could, of course, be that men are somehow genetically more creative in this sense, but this seems unlikely. What is much more likely to be true is that women are equally creative but that they are not culturally allowed to express their creativity in the same way.

Yet, it is men who make the final approach in western culture, however much women lead them to that point, and even today's fairly liberated women will often wait for the man to take the lead. That he then lays himself open to rejection, if he has misread the messages, produces a situation in which many men are permanently confused about what their women really want. Given that 'ladies' rarely say what they want, the average man has to be a kind of mind reader

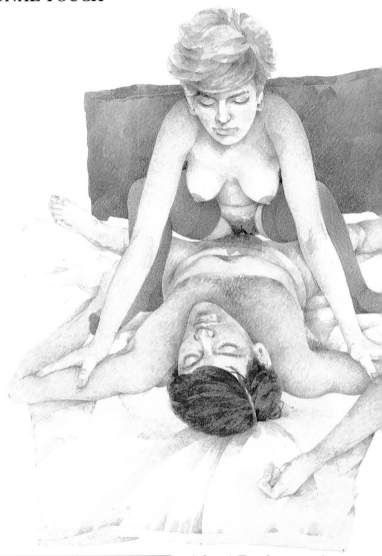

(above) For the man who has fantasies about being tied down to the bed, the woman can restrain him by holding him down and then taking a woman-on-top position to make love

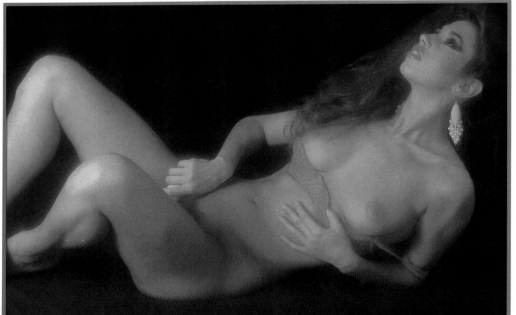

(left) If a man is particularly turned on by the thought of his partner masturbating he can ask to watch when she uses her vibrator

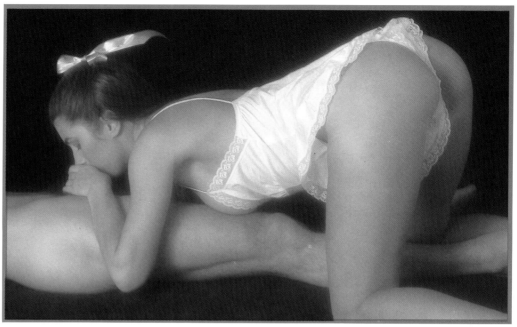

(right) Oral sex features highly among male fantasies and most men are greatly aroused by the thought of their lover bending over them to take their genitals into her mouth

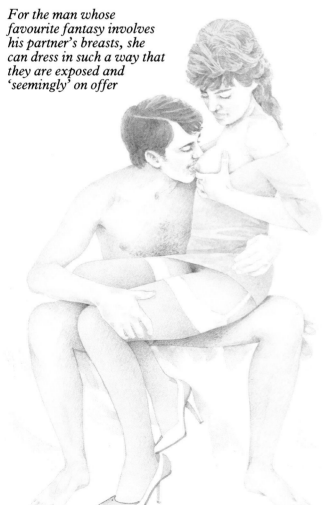

For the man whose favourite fantasy involves his partner's breasts, she can dress in such a way that they are exposed and 'seemingly' on offer

and be ready to fall flat on his face when he reads her mind wrongly.

All of this makes many men feel that women are 'impossible' to understand and to some extent they are right, if only because it can be extremely confusing to try to work out what someone wants, if they say one thing and do another often enough. Some women never express any need for sexual activity at all, yet appear to greatly enjoy it when it is offered or even 'forced' on them.

THE COMPLIANT PARTNER

So it is that in most men's fantasies the women are ready, willing and able. There is no persuasion needed here and what they, the men, do is greatly appreciated by the women in the fantasy. This is in stark contrast to many men's real-life experiences in which they cannot obtain the kind of sexual partner they would like or, if they can, she is too inhibited to do exactly what they want. And even if she does, she pretends not to have enjoyed it on the basis that 'ladies should not show too great an interest in sex for fear of appearing tarty'. It should come as no surprise then that most men fantasize about things that they cannot obtain in real life, or perhaps can only rarely do so. Women, on the contrary, fantasize most commonly about a previous romantic occasion that went very well for them.

When anyone starts to look at men's fantasies in depth, it soon becomes apparent that they are often very much more explicit and rather more extreme than most women's. Many involve animals, other men, urinary games and and so on whilst women's rarely do. It appears that men push their fantasy world to the limits much more than do women.

In fact, some are so amazing and even disgusting to

anyone other than the man himself that it seems impossible to believe that he could ever want to act them out in real life. Of course, as with women's fantasies, many, if not most, men do not want to act out their fantasies. On the contrary, to do so might reduce their value. After all, the very essence of fantasies is that everything is just perfect, which it can never be in a real life situation.

WHAT DO THEY MEAN?

Fantasy of all kinds is commonplace from the cradle onwards. The make-believe world is often much more attractive than the real one and fiction writers make their fortunes exploiting this fact.

Men daydream a lot about sex at various times of their lives just as women do. Adolescent boys can spend many long hours dreaming about a girl they lust after or love and, for a great many, such dreaming is as far as they will get either because they do not yet have the social skills to make things happen, or because they are too young to start out on the road to sexual discovery at that level.

As men age, they find it more difficult to obtain and sustain an erection. Most men over forty, for example, find that they need more stimulation if they are to obtain an erection. Some of their partners will be unwilling to extend what they will do to make this happen. For a man with this problem, there is little choice but to enrich his fantasy life, perhaps with more unusual, or at least more arousing, fantasies if his sexual life is to continue. As a result, some men in middle age start to fantasize about subjects that were previously of no interest to them.

So, often a boy will rehease in fantasy right down to the last detail what he would do in a given situation of his choice, but in many individuals the fantasy is for ever a rehearsal because real life can never be made to work in the same way.

USING FANTASY

The most common situation in which men use fantasy is when masturbating. Many adolescents, or indeed even mature men, can produce an erection just by fantasizing about their favourite subject. It can then take very little physical stimulation to give them the orgasm they want or need for relief.

Yet, there is so little research about male fantasy (female fantasy has been much more extensively studied) that it is difficult to say with any accuracy when men fantasize.

Certainly they do so during intercourse, as do many women, but for many men, if not for most, intercourse itself is sufficiently arousing and they do not usually have to use fantasy to get things going or to sustain interest.

There is little doubt that many men fantasize when making love and indeed during foreplay. Sometimes this works to their disadvantage, though, if it makes them come too quickly. Many women, on the other hand, need more stimulation of all kinds if they are to

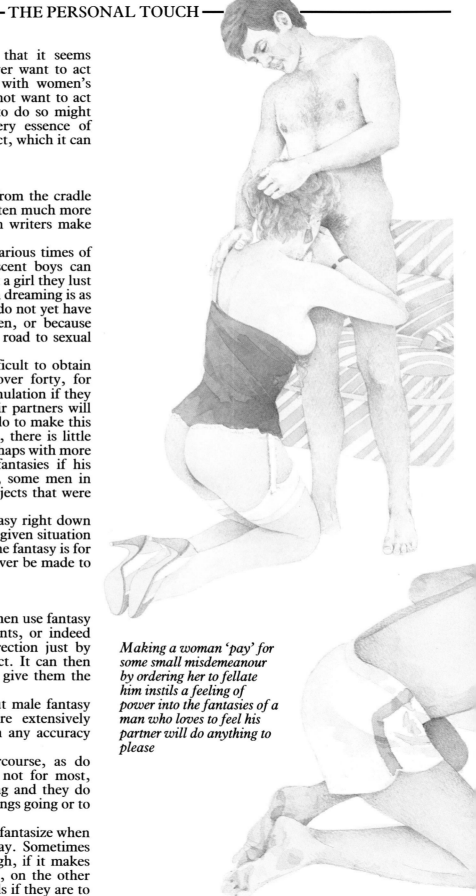

Making a woman 'pay' for some small misdemeanour by ordering her to fellate him instils a feeling of power into the fantasies of a man who loves to feel his partner will do anything to please

climax or even to enjoy intercourse without a climax, so they often call on fantasy to play a bigger role in the whole event.

SOME CLINICAL USES OF FANTASIES

Although most men have fantasies as an everyday part of their love lives and think nothing much of them in any profound sense, they can be useful for those men who have a sexual dysfunction.

Many men who have trouble with premature ejaculation, for example, will benefit greatly from masturbation training exercises.

In these, he learns to gain an erection using a favourite fantasy and then to stop stimulating his penis when it is fully erect. This makes the erection subside. He can then re-stimulate himself to get things going once more. In this way, he comes to gain control over the 'uncontrollable'. But this calls for a bank of fantasies so that he can re-awaken his limp penis many times in a row during such training.

PROBLEMS WITH ERECTION

Similarly, the man who has trouble obtaining an erection at all because he is tired, on certain drugs, is under stress, or for one of many other reasons, can, with a strong enough fantasy, make something happen when otherwise the whole sexual event would be a failure. And this is where sexual fantasy is so much more important for men than it is for women. A woman can have sex, and quite enjoyable sex, even if she is scarcely aroused. A man, on the other hand, has to be fully aroused if he is to penetrate the woman, and this can call for the use of fantasy to buttress the flagging or tired body.

Many men use their fantasies to slow themselves down or to speed themselves up during intercourse in an effort to keep pace with their partners and, provided that this does not get out of hand and become a pleasure-killer, all should be well. Far too many men today are so concerned with the pleasure of their partner that they go to all kinds of lengths to put her first. This can, however, lead to ill feeling over the months and worse if the position continued.

FETISHISM AND FANTASY

Lastly, a man who has a relatively aggressive fetish about a particular thing, say rubber, can – by being encouraged to modify his fantasies, perhaps with a

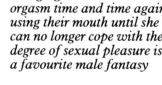

Bringing a woman to orgasm time and time again using their mouth until she can no longer cope with the degree of sexual pleasure is a favourite male fantasy

certain degree of professional help – work the problem area out of his system. The man is told to fantasize about his self-determined troublesome area until he wants to ejaculate and is advised to change the fantasy at the last minute to a more 'normal' or conventionally acceptable subject.

Slowly he can, over several weeks, reduce the amount of the rubber fantasy so that eventually he may start off thinking about it for a few moments only to replace it with his new fantasy stimulus. In time, he may then be able to rid himself of the rubber fantasy altogether, as, perhaps with the help of his partner, he replaces the old fantasy entirely with the new.

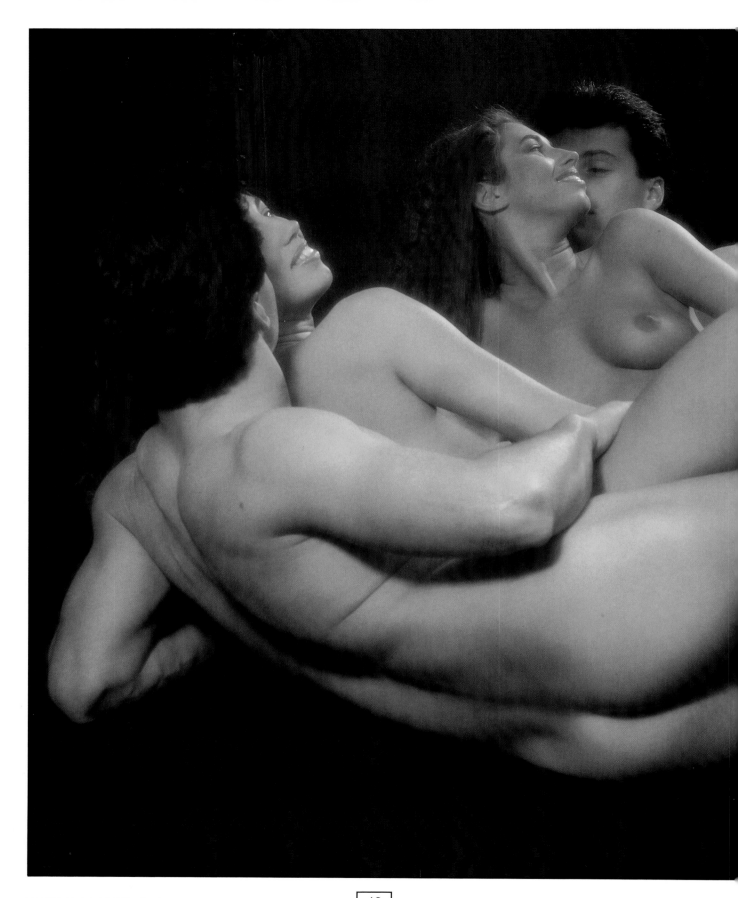

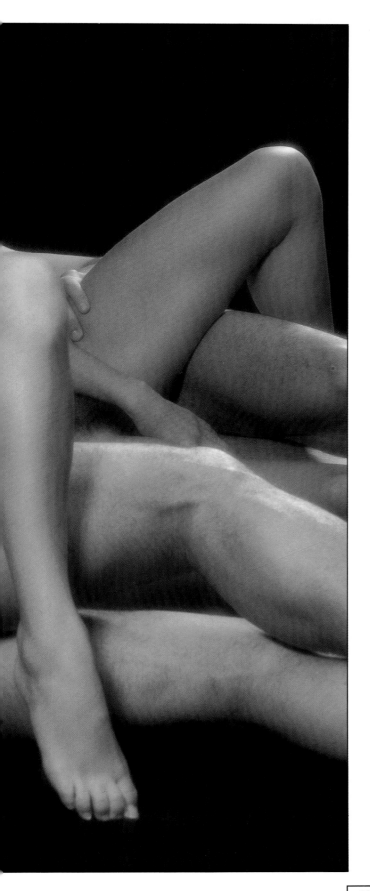

CREATIVE LOVEMAKING

Sex can be passionate, gentle, fun, exciting, soothing, inventive – but there is no reason why it shouldn't always be fulfilling. Taking a fresh look at your lovemaking techniques can open up new avenues to pleasure, and keep that initial thrill of romance alive in your relationship beyond the early days and into the years ahead

MAKING SEX MEMORABLE

Familiarity can be a boon to good lovemaking, but, from time to time, it pays to vary your sexual routine and add a little magic to your love life

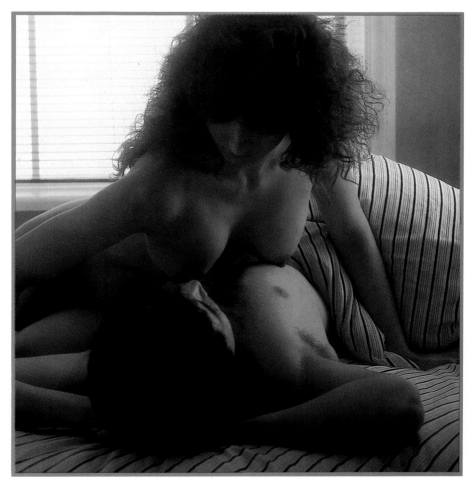

Even in the safety of the bedroom, sex can be made memorable for any couple prepared to be a little adventurous or willing to talk about their needs with one another

After a couple have been making love for a few months, they tend to settle into a sexual routine. There is nothing wrong with this. Good sex is about experimenting and finding what suits you both best and, through this, knowing how best to give pleasure to your partner.

Although in a perfect world sex would be memorable every time we made love, unfortunately, for most couples, the routine may mean good, satisfying and familiar sex, but the memory is probably lost by the following day.

A MILESTONE

Everyone has a memory of that one time or times when sex with their partner was so special that it had an almost magical quality about it. The setting was both romantic and erotic, the foreplay was fantastically arousing and the orgasms, when they came, were simultaneous and almost breathtaking in their intensity. That kind of sex becomes a milestone in any couple's life together although they probably rarely refer to it. These occasions are special providing the kind of material to us, towards which we naturally aspire.

BY ACCIDENT – NOT BY DESIGN

The chances are that it came about by accident rather than design which makes its magical quality all the more complicated to understand. There is no reason, however, why sex should not be more memorable more often; all you need is a little extra effort.

WHAT MAKES SEX MEMORABLE?

What makes one lovemaking episode special rather than another with the same partner can be difficult to explain. What is certain, though, is that it has less to do with one partner's sexual technique than the mood which preceded it. Even the most sexually experienced and athletic partner can fail to give the right sensations to his or her partner if the mood is wrong.

THE RIGHT MOOD

The back of the car, a deserted beach or the comfort of one's own bedroom can all have magical qualities for sex if the mood is right. Creating such an atmosphere after a couple has been together for some time needs preparation and imagination – and it requires time. Lovemaking in a hurry may be fine on some occasions, but the sensations that bring us to the brink of a unique orgasm and beyond usually demand that time is spent on us – not just on kissing and caressing, but in the words we use to each other, the small looks and glances we exchange and the amount of loving attention we pay to our partner. Familiarity may breed better lovemaking, technically, but pre-sexual foreplay – the period of courtship sometimes called the honeymoon period – is something that is sadly forgotten by many couples after they have been together for a little while.

AFTER A WHILE

Yet the couple who have been together for a period of time and who have become used to each other's sexual likes and dislikes are, in fact, in a good position to make sex memorable for each other. This is because they already know each other's sexual preferences and so are in less danger of accidentally doing something, or suggesting something, that the other finds sexually distasteful. Because of that, they can exploit their own situation to create memorable sex for each other.

IMAGINATIVE FOREPLAY

The quality of foreplay can make or break a lovemaking session. Treat it perfunctorily and the sex can all too easily become ordinary and predictable. Pay attention to it and use your imagination and the experience becomes almost totally unique.

But before foreplay, making sex memorable for your partner involves deciding on what they want and like best and then putting it into action. Making a

lovemaking episode linger on in the memory involves putting yourself in your partner's place for a moment and then creating the atmosphere that you know instinctively be right.

FOR HER

Decide what atmosphere you wish to create. It is worth noting that most research tends to show that women are more influenced by the place in which they make love than are men. So if your partner loves romantic, candlelit evenings for two at home, prepare

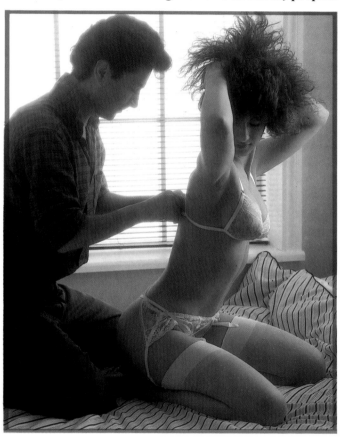

one for her. If she likes making love in unusual places, do your best to accommodate her. If she likes flowers or small presents then give them to her. And if she likes you to dress in a particular way, then do so.

Concentrate on giving her everything that she wants during the whole time that you have set aside for lovemaking, down to the smallest detail. It is likely that when you first started making love with her you were 'on your best behaviour'. You were attentive, you listened to everything she said – in short, you behaved like a lover should.

There may have been a selfish element to all this in the sense that you realized that lovemaking would be more pleasant for you – and more certain – if you behaved in this way. But whatever the reasons, it is a comparatively simple matter to re-create this behaviour.

FOR HIM

Contrary to the opinion of many 'experts', most men are no less influenced by mood when it comes to lovemaking. It is just that their sexual parameters are slightly different. As women tend to be more influenced by the setting and the 'romantic' trimmings, men tend to be more visually stimulated by their partner. It is your body, and often the way you are dressed, that can make sex memorable for him. For the woman who wants to make sex memorable for her partner – as well as herself – it may make sense to dress for him periodically. So if he fancies you as a 'tart', dress like one.

Similarly with sexual behaviour – if you are going to dress like a whore for him, behave like one. Tease him almost unmercifully. Use your body to tantalize him. If you decide to wear no underwear to excite him, tell him that this is what you have done. Treat sex unselfishly, concentrating on making it memorable for him and, by so doing, make it memorable for yourself.

ORGASM
One or both partners' orgasm is generally the aim of lovemaking but often the most memorable sex can be achieved by bringing each other to the verge of orgasm rather than allowing each other to come straight away. Sometimes orgasm can be all the sweeter and more powerful if you have nearly achieved it only to subside and then be brought up to it again. But to avoid

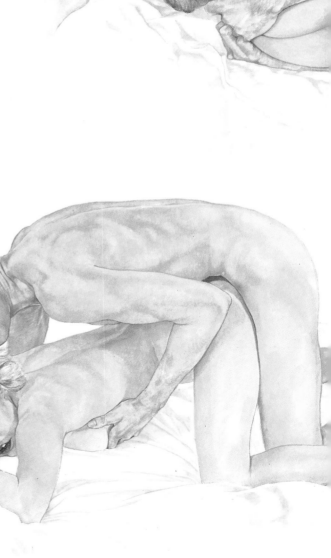

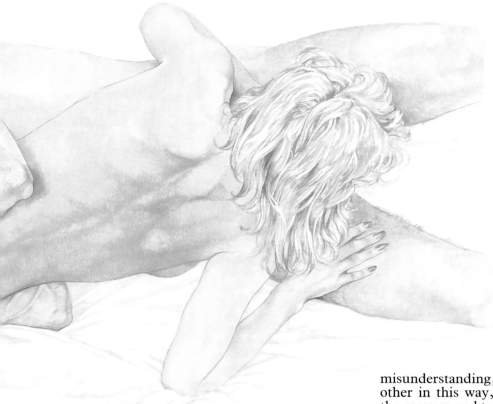

Some women find it highly arousing when their partner kisses their perineum — the classic '69' position allows you to do this and also to stimulate the vulva area

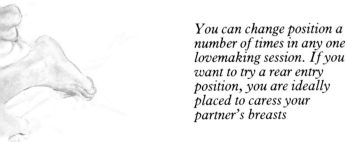

You can change position a number of times in any one lovemaking session. If you want to try a rear entry position, you are ideally placed to caress your partner's breasts

misunderstanding, if you do decide to 'tease' each other in this way, tell each other beforehand. Then, the caresses and techniques that follow can be repeated and expanded on time and again.

HIM – FOR HER

To bring your partner to the brink of orgasm make undressing her a lingering experience and combine it with creative kissing and caressing. Take time removing each garment, always using your hands to run up and down her back, her legs and her stomach. Nibble her feet and calves and behind her knees. Encourage her to stretch out and abandon herself to you.

When she is totally naked, use oil all over her but do not touch her breasts or vulva. Instead, lightly brush over them as you caress her less erogenous zones. Alternate between using your fingers and the palm of your hands. Use your lips as well.

INTIMATE CARESSING
When you do start to caress her breasts, pour oil directly on to them and knead it in. Then use the tip of your penis to trace a path around each nipple. If she tries to touch you, restrain her. Then use oil on her vulva with the other hand, first of all circling it before gently using a finger on her clitoris using slow and delicate movements. When she is ready, insert as many fingers as she likes into her vagina and use the thumb of your hand on her clitoris. Do not allow her to come at this stage.

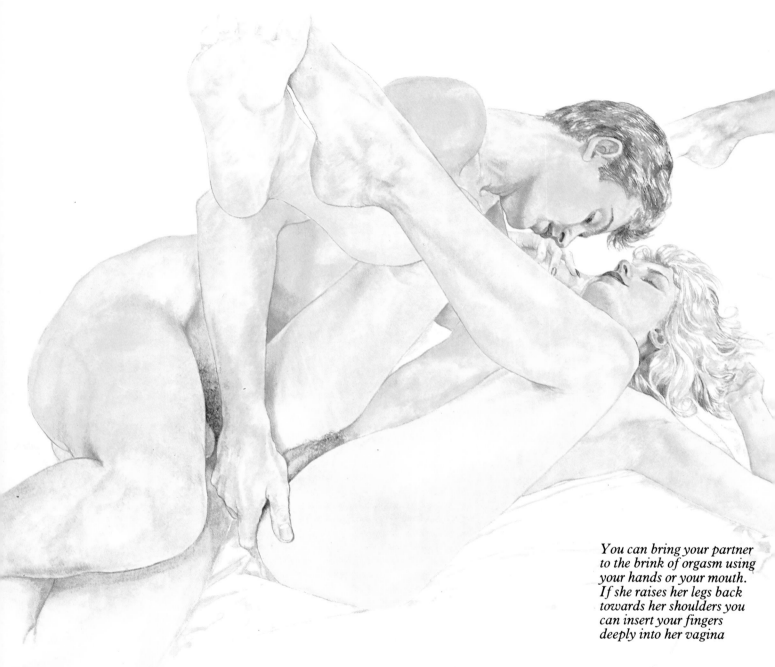

You can bring your partner to the brink of orgasm using your hands or your mouth. If she raises her legs back towards her shoulders you can insert your fingers deeply into her vagina

USING A VIBRATOR

Apart from your own body, a vibrator is one of the most versatile and variable sex aids for a woman. There are a number of ways you can use it on her, but for the purpose of making sex memorable do not use it to bring her to orgasm, only to the brink. Use it on her breasts and her buttocks as well as her vulva. If she likes it, insert the tip into her anus as well, although remember not to put it in her vagina afterwards as this may transfer anal bacteria.

Vary the speed setting as you alternate using it inside her and on her clitoris. Make sure, as well, that you keep your other hand and mouth busy elsewhere to please her.

HER – FOR HIM

Men love to be caressed and fussed over as much as women. The only difference is that, because they are more genitally orientated, they tend to require less time to become aroused. So although the quality of

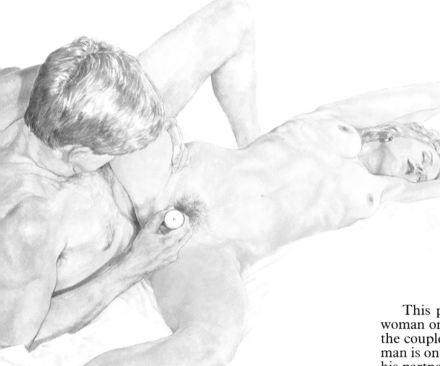

Used creatively, a vibrator can give your partner exquisite sensations. Use it to massage her thighs and the area around her genitals before using it directly on her clitoris

This position is usually best approached with the woman on top, although it can be sensually relaxing if the couple lay side by side. It can be satisfactory if the man is on top as well, but the temptation to thrust into his partner's mouth is often too great for some men. If the woman likes this then that is fine but, as a general rule, it is best for the woman to control the movements of her mouth on the man's penis rather than vice versa. In any event, take up a position that is comfortable for you both.

THE WOMAN'S APPROACH

Mutual oral sex is highly erotic if your partner lies back on the bed and you squat over his mouth, facing away from him, and give him a full genital kiss on the lips using the vulva.

Remember that your partner will find this highly arousing as well, not only for the sensations that he is giving you, but because of the view he has of your buttocks.

Lean slowly forward and rest on the bed with one elbow. Take the root of his penis into your other hand and direct it into your mouth. Use long strokes, taking it as deeply into your mouth as you comfortably can and alternate this with licking the tip of his penis and sucking on it. All the time, remember to move your buttocks and direct his tongue on to your clitoris. If you like him to lick your perineum and anus, then all you need to do is adjust your position slightly.

Remember that you are in control when orgasm takes place. Most men will find this position so highly arousing that, if you increase the pace too frantically, your partner may come too soon. So do not be tempted to move your head too quickly or to suck too hard.

When you feel your own orgasm approaching, is it

arousal should be memorable for him, it should not take too long or be too intense, otherwise your partner will come too soon which may be fine for him but not so good for you.

Use your hands in conjunction with your body to caress him. Trace a path along his back from his feet to his neck with your hands and bring your breasts along behind. Use your nipples on his buttocks – perhaps teasing his perineum with them.

Then turn him over and pour oil on to his stomach and the tops of his legs. Rub it firmly in and then pour some more directly on to the tip of his penis and gently rub it in with both hands.

PERFECT ORGASMS

A session of lovemaking may last anything from a few minutes to half an hour or more. It may involve one or both partners coming once or several times.

But, whatever position or lovemaking technique you choose, remember that it can always be changed if the mood changes. And orgasm may not necessarily be genitally induced – it could always be oral.

THE '69' POSITION
The '69' position can be a mind-blowing way to achieve simultaneous and memorable orgasms – for both partners – if it is approached in the right way.

time to increase the momentum. Move your hand up and down his penis as you use your lips, tongue and mouth to bring him to orgasm. Increase the pace and literally rub yourself over his mouth, directing him to use it on the places you like best. Press your breasts into his stomach and move your mouth as furiously as you can.

THE MAN'S APPROACH

Accept that from this position, the woman will control the pace of lovemaking and try to coincide your orgasm with hers. When she squats over your face use your tongue as creatively as you can. Start off by licking her clitoris and then try taking it between your lips and teeth and sucking on it. Be guided by what she wants. If you know she likes to have her perineum licked then do so. Do not keep your hands idle either. Use them to part her vaginal lips and pop your tongue inside her.

Transfer your fingers inside her – put in as many as she likes and use your tongue on her clitoris. Show that she is giving you pleasure by thrusting upwards into her mouth and responding to the rhythm that she creates. Concentrate your efforts on holding back your own orgasm until she comes.

POSITIONS

For penis-in-vagina sex, the actual position you use is not too important. The golden rule is to choose one you both like and use it as creatively and imaginatively as you can. Also do not regard this one position as the only one you can use. Be prepared to swap over while you are making love. This is important, because

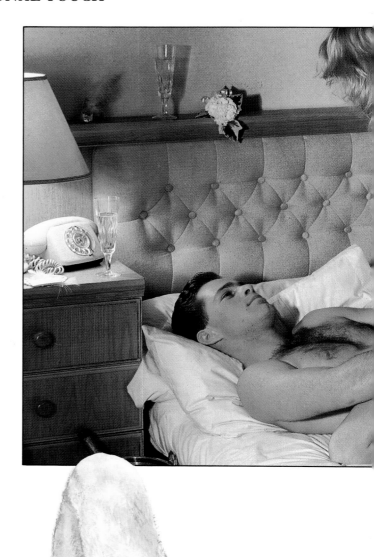

A change from more usual 'man-on-top' positions can soon improve any couple's sex life. With the reverse missionary position the woman can take on a more dominant role in lovemaking while her partner can control her thrusting movements by wrapping his leg over her bottom

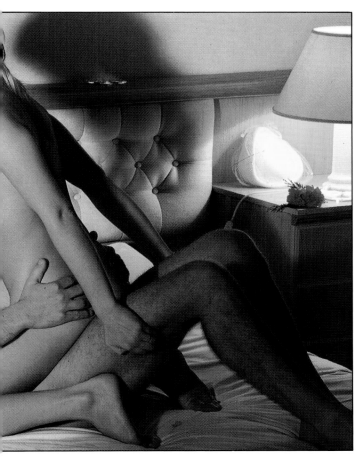

By positioning herself on top, a woman can watch her lover's response as she sets the rhythm of their lovemaking

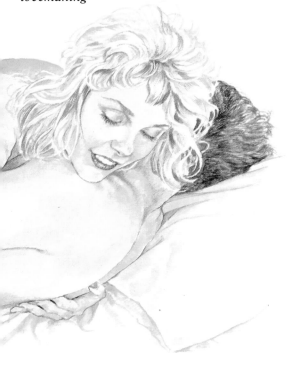

moods and needs can change during any individual session of lovemaking. The woman may suddenly want to take on a more dominant role, for example, or she may want to be penetrated from behind. Equally, the man may relish a change to a more aggressive or passive style of lovemaking after a while. All that is important – and the loving couple will recognize this – is that they are in tune with each other's needs. So whatever position you choose, concentrate on sexual movement and rhythm.

Try to ancitipate each other's needs. In a man-on-top position, this means the man controlling his thrusting and trying to control the timing of his own orgasm. For the woman, it means knowing when and how to move her body in response to her partner's movements.

And for both of them, lovemaking can be considerably enhanced if attention is paid to sideways movements as well as thrusting. For the man, the sight and sensations of the woman moving from side to side as she rotates the bottom part of her body can be highly arousing. Similarly, for the woman the sight of the man as he moves his hips from side to side can be equally stimulating.

RHYTHM AND TIMING

Good intercourse is all about rhythm and timing as well. The most determined thrusting can all be to no avail if the rhythm and timing are wrong. For perfect lovemaking, try and keep the rhythm in response to whoever is taking the initiative; ideally, one should be in control. So if the pace is slow, respond in the same way and, as it speeds up, concentrate on timing your own response. Lovemaking, performed like this, can almost become an art form as the couple rises and falls, penetrates and withdraws – and finally comes – together.

THE G-SPOT ORGASM

For the woman who has a sensitive G spot, lovemaking can be particularly special if she achieves a G-spot-induced orgasm as well as a clitoral one. And for the man to witness and be the means of her achieving it, as well as having a powerful orgasm himself, this can be truly memorable.

The woman should kneel down on the bed and put her face down on the pillow and offer her buttocks to you as high as she can with her legs wide apart – the idea being that when you penetrate her and start thrusting you will be able to hit her G spot every time. She will be able to adjust the position so that you do this. She should keep one hand free to stimulate her clitoris. Enter her gently and start thrusting slowly at first. Encourage her to start stimulating herself and slowly increase the tempo. By the time you sense that her orgasm is approaching, you should be going as fast as you can. Use your hands to part her buttocks, perhaps playfully slapping them if that is what she enjoys or, if she likes it, pop a finger in her anus at the moment of orgasm.

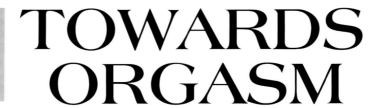

TOWARDS ORGASM

The journey towards orgasm can be full of the most exquisite sensations when masturbation or oral sex are used to heighten the level of arousal

Foreplay does not finish when intercourse begins. From time to time, there is a middle stage where masturbation and oral sex have an important part to play – either as part of arousal or as an alternative to conventional intercourse.

BE CREATIVE

Sexually, our hands and mouths are the most versatile parts of our bodies. We use them to caress and touch, to kiss and lick – even tickle. Our brain stores up knowledge of our partner's special needs and during foreplay relays messages to our hands and mouths – as well as our genitals – which readily respond. For the giver, the unique pleasure of exploring a partner's body is only surpassed by being the means of providing them with their orgasm.

And for the receiver, the knowledge that the hands and lips can be trusted to probe and explore the genitals also brings a unique pleasure that only comes from familiarity and intimate knowledge of our body and its special needs. The ability of a skilled lover always to find the spot that gives pleasure and maintain a rhythm that their partner can respond to is one of the true bonuses of a loving relationship.

THE ADVANTAGES

Both masturabation and oral sex can be used to good effect in an established relationship, not just for the mutual pleasure they provide but also when things are going wrong – perhaps when intercourse is difficult through illness, during the late stages of pregnancy

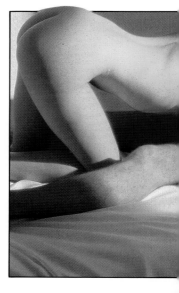

Both men and women can use their mouths and tongues to stimulate their partners to the edge of orgasm – and beyond

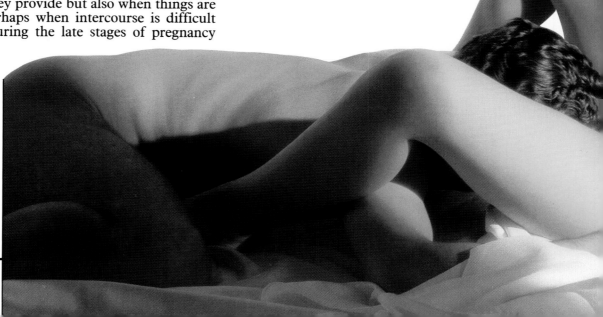

and immediately afterwards, or merely if either partner feels uncertain about sex for any reason.

Masturbation, particularly, needs to have its rightful place. Even in the most loving and satisfying relationships, it does not stop once a full sex life is established. One clinical survey suggested that masturbation is even more likely to take place when a couple have a satisfying sex life – perhaps, the more sex you have, the more you want.

Equally with oral sex. When the mouth is brought into play and is used with unique intimacy, mimicking as it can the movements of a vagina or the penis, it can prove to be a love-gift of unparalleled intimacy. And if penetration is not possible for some reason – if the man fails to achieve an erection or he has come too soon and wants to bring his partner to orgasm – the mouth, as an alternative to genital intercourse, has no peer.

TIMING

Perhaps the greatest advantage of shared masturbation and oral sex is that they can be used as a kind of sexual timing device. Most couples, rightly or wrongly, see simultaneous orgasm as the pinnacle of their love-making. If the man, for example, is prone to come too soon during conventional intercourse, he can use his hands and lips to bring his partner to the brink of orgasm before he penetrates her. He should then be able to time his own orgasm to coincide with hers.

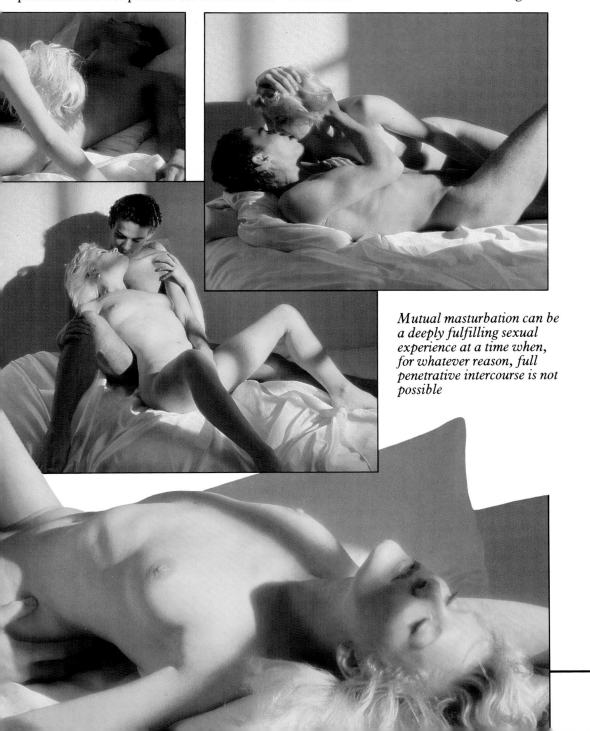

Mutual masturbation can be a deeply fulfilling sexual experience at a time when, for whatever reason, full penetrative intercourse is not possible

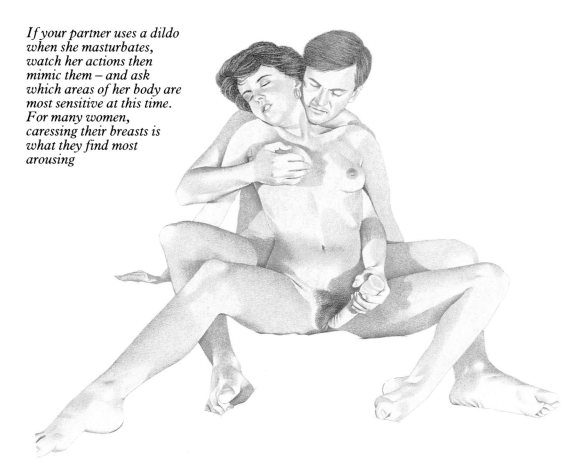

If your partner uses a dildo when she masturbates, watch her actions then mimic them – and ask which areas of her body are most sensitive at this time. For many women, caressing their breasts is what they find most arousing

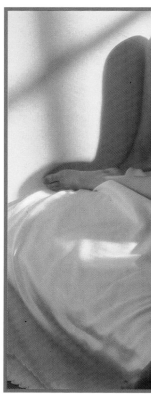

Similarly, the partner of a man who, perhaps as he becomes older, finds that his orgasm takes longer to build up than it used to, can use her hands or mouth to bring him to the verge of orgasm thus enabling her climax to coincide with his.

And for the woman who wants a second orgasm, her mouth will almost invariably be able to re-arouse all but the most reluctant lover. Not for nothing is oral sex called a reviver of the dead.

LEARNING THROUGH MASTURBATION

It is from masturbation that we first discover what gives us pleasure sexually. We learn how our genitals and our bodies repond to touch and we learn how best to bring ourselves to orgasm. From that experience, we are then able to tell another person – our partner – what we like best. In the sexual arena, we are always the best tutors as to how we should be pleased.

And, as in almost everything we do, we learn from imitation. Through watching how a partner brings him or herself to orgasm, we can learn how best to pleasure them.

So ask what your partner likes best, get them to masturbate in front of you and imitate their actions later. And try not to judge your present partner from previous ones.

By all means experiment with what you have learned from earlier lovers, but always be prepared to

shelve earlier knowledge in favour of new wisdom. It is the person you are with at a particular time that you want to please – not someone else.

HANDWORK

It is assumed that you are familiar with your lover's body and that you have brought them to orgasm with your hands and fingers as well as through conventional intercourse. The purpose of good – or advanced – handwork is to improve and enhance the quality of your partner's orgasm for them. It is also assumed that you will have used creative and imaginative foreplay on their non-genital areas to bring them to a state of readiness. As a result of this, you can use your hands either to bring them to orgasm, or to the brink of it, before intercourse takes place.

CHOOSE THE RIGHT POSITION

You may choose to vary the position you use from time to time, but the main consideration is that both of you are comfortable. Your partner should feel relaxed and at ease, but your own comfort is almost equally important – otherwise you are going to find that you are constantly changing positions. So, get as close to your partner's genitals as you can.

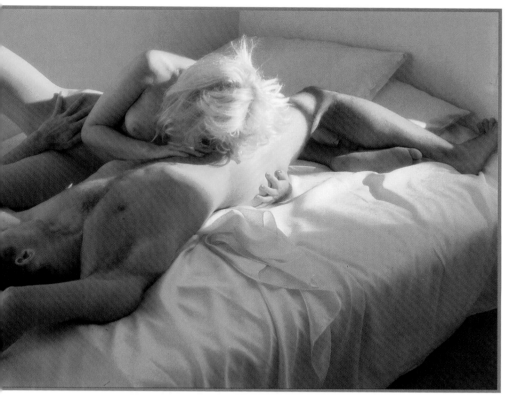

(left) While your partner takes your genitals into her mouth, you should not ignore her needs. Gently caress her stomach or breasts to arouse her while she pleases you

(below) Whether sitting up or lying down, kissing your partner while gently masturbating her will make her feel more relaxed and reassured

nipples caressed as they are being masturbated – some may like them squeezed. Others may like their bottom or anus teased – some may like their lover to put a finger inside.

Similarly, a man may like his testes and scrotum massaged as well as his penis and many men greatly enjoy the woman lighly scratching their perineum. You will know from watching your partner what their special needs are, so be sure that you remember to cater for them.

MAKE IT GOOD

Above all, make it memorable. The setting and the mood should be right and the temperature warm enough. Make your hands all embracing – allow your partner to know that your intentions are to use your hands to bring them to an explosive orgasm. Ensure that there is no hurry – and be prepared to change tack if you sense that this is what they want.

An orgasm approaches and if your partner appears to want intercourse – or for you to use your mouth – be prepared to do so. Through this versatility and unselfishness you will also increase your own pleasure when it is your 'turn'.

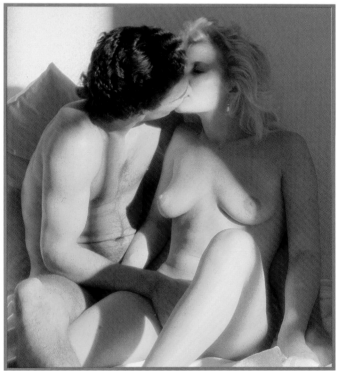

BE AWARE OF SPECIAL NEEDS

Although the result of masturbation is usually orgasm, different people have such varied requirements that the advanced lover must be sensitive to the other's needs. Many women, for example like their breasts or

HIM TO HER

Because women's sexual needs are so variable, many will prefer to be stimulated in different ways. What follows is a suggestion that is open to many variations.

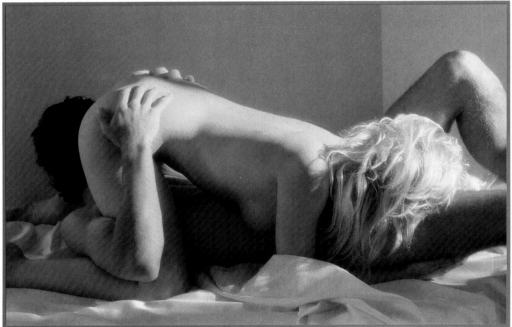

While licking and sucking your partner's penis, gently move your genitals over his face. His mouth and tongue can then caress and penetrate your clitoris and vagina

Having kissed, caressed and massaged her, carefully avoiding her genitals, place a couple of pillows in the centre of the bed – or on the carpet if she prefers – and get her to lay across them so that the pillows are directly underneath her stomach. Ensure that she is comfortable.

Her bottom should now be raised high and her vulva exposed. Ask her to part her legs and then apply liberal amounts of massage or baby oil to her buttocks so that it seeps down the cleft between them and on to her vulva.

Use both hands to rub the oil into her bottom. Then, with one hand still kneading her buttocks, gently apply the oil around her vulva, but without touching her clitoris yet. Use the other hand to alternate between a circular sweeping motion on her buttocks and rubbing her thighs, keeping up a light yet insistent motion in the whole area around her vaginal lips. As the tempo increases, but not the pressure, move to her clitoris and start to massage it delicately with your fingers.

As you feel her becoming more aroused, you can alternate between using your fingers and the palm of your hand in order to provide a different, heightened type of sensation for her.

As her clitoris enlarges, keep on caressing it and 'dip' a finger of your other hand into her vagina. Depending on how receptive she is and what she wants, one finger may not be sufficient – be guided by how many you know she needs.

Now, with one hand directly stimulating her clitoris, start to caress her vagina.

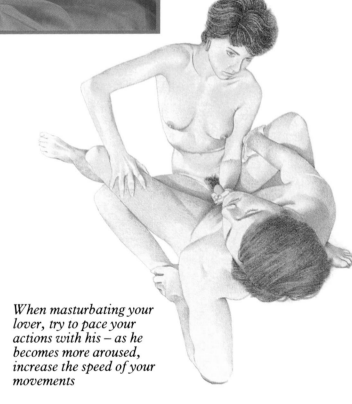

When masturbating your lover, try to pace your actions with his – as he becomes more aroused, increase the speed of your movements

EXPLORE HER VAGINA

You may be able to feel your partner's cervix at the top end of her vagina with your fingers. Some women greatly enjoy having this caressed. If she does, carry on massaging this, or you can move on to her ovaries – at the sides of the top of the vagina. Also, if your partner has a sensitive G spot (on the front wall of her vagina), make sure that your movements inside her vagina stimulate this as well. This should double the intensity of her orgasm when it comes.

In any event, start to use your fingers to produce thrusting movements inside her vagina, increasing the tempo all the time – rather as you would if you were using your penis. When she approaches orgasm, increase the rhythm still further. When her orgasm comes and she moves her body, try to keep your own rhythm in time with hers. Be sensitive to the pace of her orgasm and concentrate on making it the most explosive she has ever had. And as her sensations subside, slow your movements down before kissing and cuddling her.

HER TO HIM

Many women think that they can do just about anything to a man's penis to bring him to orgasm. To some extent this is true, but if the quality of his orgasm is to reach its maximum potential, it pays to give as much attention to what you know he likes and, if necessary, expand and try to improve on it.

After massaging him with oil, lie him down on the bed or carpet – some men may like to be restrained by having their hands lightly tied to the bed posts or

something similar, but this is optional – and turn him over on to his front. Apply oil to his buttocks and vigorously massage them, pressing them together. Use your fingers to massage oil into his perineum using featherlight strokes. Remember that at this stage, you are teasing him rather than hurrying him.

When he has an erection turn him over and pour the oil directly on the tip of his penis – this will greatly excite him. Then, choose a position for yourself that he likes. If he likes to have you squatting over his face pressing your vulva down on to his lips, then do so. But remember, most men will find a position like this highly arousing which in turn will increase the speed at which they have their orgasm.

USE BOTH HANDS

Now, rub the oil gently into his testes and scrotum, perhaps lightly brushing against his penis as you do this. Then, in order not to tease him too much, move on to the final stage.

Use both hands, rub the oil into the shaft of his penis. Go very slowly at first – using a circular rubbing motion on each side of the penis. To increase his sensations still further, perhaps use your tongue to lick the tip of his penis. Then, as gradually as you can, increase the speed and the pressure at which your hands are working. This should be almost imperceptible.

As his orgasm approaches, increase the speed and pressure as much as is comfortable – men vary in how much is desirable – and as he begins to ejaculate, increase the speed still further. Imagine that you are squeezing out every last drop of seminal fluid.

The golden rule is to always keep one step ahead of

Do not limit your attention only to your partner's vagina – many women like to be kissed or have their stomach caressed while they are being masturbated

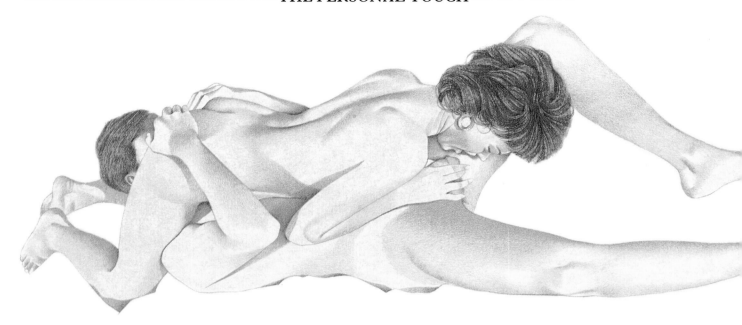

his movements. As his body starts to move up and down, so should your hand movements become even more insistent. Then, as the power of the ejaculation decreases, begin to slow down, releasing the pressure.

MOUTHWORK

Oral sex, for most of those who practise it, is delightful – the pleasures of giving equalling those of receiving. It is sometimes seen by couples as a one-sided affair, but there can be as much pleasure for the person who takes the other's genitals in their mouth as there is for the receiver. Remember, though, that it is usually the final stage of oral sex – when the penis is taken into the mouth, or the man uses his lips and tongue on the clitoris – that tends to receive most attention. In fact, good oral sex is concerned with the use of the mouth, lips and tongue all over the other person's body.

FOR HER

For the couple who regularly use oral sex, making it more memorable for her can be achieved by using a vibrator or dildo as well as your lips and tongue.

To do this, it is best for the woman to lie back on the bed as she would if you were going to make love to her in the missionary position. And if the vibrator is to be used, it is best used in earlier foreplay – perhaps to stimulate her breasts and buttocks – rather than being brought out towards the end of a lovemaking session.

Open her legs as wide as is comfortable for her and take up a position in between them that is comfortable for you. It is a good idea to use a couple of pillows underneath her bottom so that she is then 'offering' herself to you.

Start by nuzzling into her vulva and kiss her pubic hair. Then gently use both hands to part her vulval lips and run your tongue lightly around them. Suck the small lips gently, then lick the area around the vagina as well as immediately beneath it. Poke your tongue into her vagina and push it gently in and out. Then, using your hands to open up her vagina, kiss and lick all around her clitoris and taking care to go gently on the tip itself, which some women find extremely sensitive. Keep a regular rhythm going and spend as much time as is necessary on each part of her before turning your attention fully to her clitoris.

Now, as you lick her clitoris, is the time to use the vibrator. Insert the vibrator into her vagina and, using the lowest setting, aim to find her G spot. It may help if you encourage her to put her legs over your shoulders at this stage. Then, still using your tongue, slowly increase the speed setting on the vibrator and begin to use thrusting movements as you would with your penis. You should be able to sense when her orgasm is coming and increase the pace accordingly. Vary the sweep on her clitoris with your tongue and increase the pace as her climax approaches, and concentrate on hitting her G spot with each stroke of the vibrator. As her orgasm subsides, gently withdraw the vibrator and softly lick around her vulval area. Caress and kiss her. If she is ready for another orgasm, you can then penetrate her from this position.

FOR HIM

For many men, having oral sex performed on them is almost preferable to conventional intercourse. This is partly because his partner's mouth is more versatile than her vagina and is thus able to provide unique sensations for a man. Also, psychologically, the man may feel that his penis is being worshipped, which

(left) In the 69 position, both partners can experience the delights of oral sex – be sensitive to your lover's level of arousal and lighten your touch if he appears to be reaching orgasm more quickly than you

A man's tongue and lips can be ideal 'sex aids' when used to arouse his partner – the tongue can be used to mimic the actions of a penis, but in a much gentler way, and kisses planted on the perineum can be highly arousing

Use both your hands and your mouth to arouse your partner. Take as much of his penis as you feel comfortable with into your mouth – if you take too much you will gag – and use your hands to stimulate the root of his penis or to caress his testes. If he likes it, you can also caress his buttocks or his anus

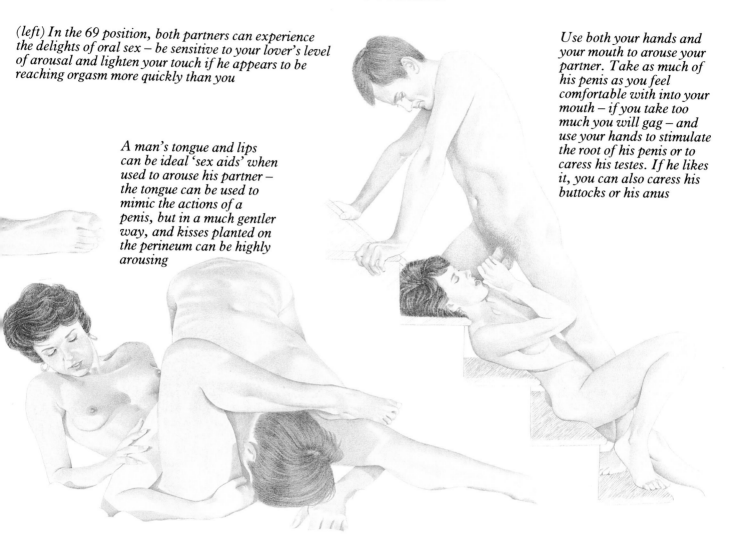

makes him feel highly desirable in a sexual sense.

To give your partner a slightly different orgasm while using your lips and tongue on his penis, you can try using your fingers to stimulate his G spot – his prostate – if he likes this. Alternatively, you can concentrate on keeping your hands busy elsewhere on his body.

POSITIONS

There are a number of positions in which fellatio can be performed, from the man standing and the woman kneeling before him, or both partners lying down, to the athletic and the bizarre.

For the purposes of achieving a memorable orgasm for your partner, one of the lying-down positions is probably best – perhaps with your partner's head supported on a pillow so that he is best able to see what you are doing.

Make sure that you are both comfortable, then take his penis into the palm of your hand and moisten it with saliva. Now, insert the head of the penis into your mouth and take it in as deeply as you feel is comfortable for you. Move your mouth up and down

so that the penis moves in and out of your mouth, sucking as you do so. Put one hand around the root of his penis and move it slowly up and down as well. Alternate this between licking the penis tip and running your tongue along its shaft.

MASSAGE HIS 'G SPOT'

As the tempo increases, use a little KY jelly and pop your finger into his anus to find his prostate gland – he may need to bring his legs up to enable you to do this and you should take care of long fingernails – all the time using your mouth on his penis in continual fellatio as you do so.

Now, keeping an insistent rhythm as you suck his penis, use your finger to massage his prostate. As you sense his orgasm approaching, take his penis as deeply into your mouth as you can and, if you are happy doing so, swallow his semen.

Alternatively, withdraw your mouth and use your free hand to bring him to orgasm, perhaps with him coming over your breasts or any other part of your body. Then, when he has come, lovingly lick the end of his penis until his erection has subsided.

COME TOGETHER

Climaxing together is not essential in order to make sex enjoyable, but when it does happen, it can make lovemaking memorable – for both partners

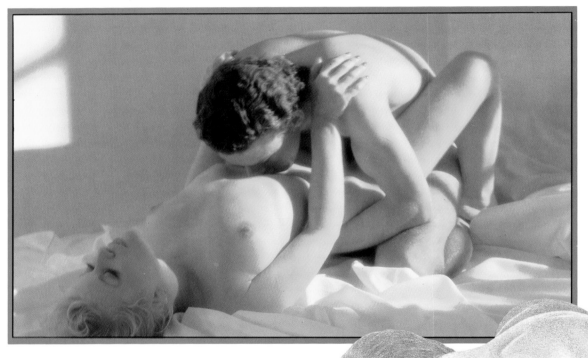

Most, if not all, lovers expect – or at least would like – every lovemaking session to end in orgasm for both partners – and preferably at the same time. For many couples this often proves difficult to achieve, yet, with care and sensitivity, simultaneous orgasm is well within the compass of most loving couples who best know each other's unique and individual needs.

TIMING
Generally, a woman takes longer to reach orgasm than a man. Even given the most perfect lovemaking technique from her partner, she is going to require more creative foreplay than him. This is not to say that the quality of the orgasm cannot be greatly enhanced for a man depending on the quality of arousal, but left to their own devices, most men could probably achieve orgasm in less minute and probably less.

If the time is right, this may happen for a woman some of the time, but the chances are she is going to take longer. The advanced lover knows this and increases the quality of her arousal before intercourse takes place.

COMPLICATIONS

The situation is further complicated by the fact that a number of women are perfectly able to reach orgasm through masturbation, oral sex or by using a vibrator, but cannot come during conventional intercourse. The secret for them is choose one of the positions where the woman is best able to stimulate her clitoris – generally a woman-on-top position – or one where the man can do it for her as they make love. Then, simultaneous orgasm should, and can, be possible.

In any event, the golden rule for the couple who want to come together lies in the timing. Of course, getting the timing right is not that simple – if it were, every couple would always come when they wanted and how they wanted. Some women are multi-orgasmic, some only rarely have orgasms and the quality and nature of a man's orgasm can vary quite surprisingly, too.

WHO TAKES CHARGE?

In most lovemaking sessions, it is important that one partner takes overall control and is the 'doer'. This can be done in a number of ways.

If the man feels his own orgasm approaching without any sign of his partner's, he can change the tempo of lovemaking. He can either control the pace of intercourse by keeping his thrusting to a minimum while caressing his partner, or he can withdraw his penis and bring her to the brink of orgasm with his fingers, mouth, or vibrator before entering her again. The lover who is in tune with his partner will know, also, whether a change of position is called for and will adapt accordingly. Eventually, it should be possible to make love to one's partner almost intuitively, allowing pleasure to take its full course.

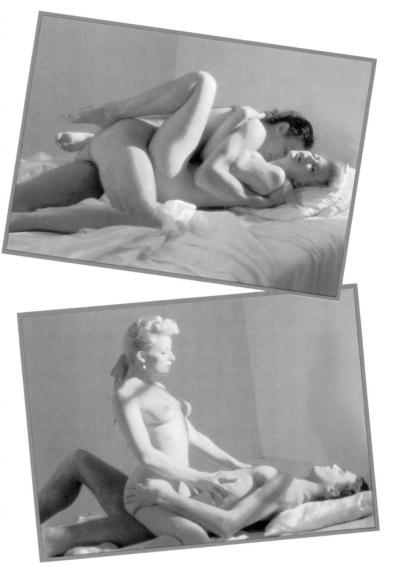

(above) Experimenting with different positions during lovemaking can help couples match the pace of their orgasms

(left) Though not vital to an enjoyable sex life, coming together can be a deeply satisfying shared experience

(right) Penetration will not be as deep if you enter your partner from behind while lying on your sides, but it will allow you to stimulate her clitoris at the same time

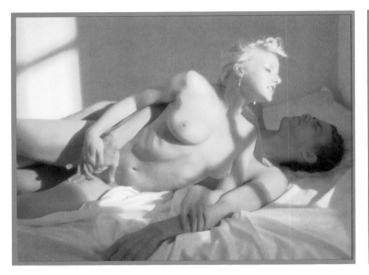
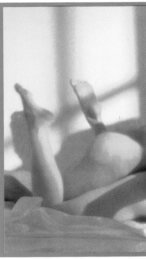

(middle) If you ask your partner to lie on her front you can thrust more deeply as you penetrate from behind

WOMAN IN CHARGE

Similarly, a woman who feels her own orgasm will take longer than her partner's can take control and use her body to slow him down. She can do this by keeping his arousal down to a minimum while increasing the level of her own. Then, by choosing a position where she dictates the pace of intercourse, she can bring herself towards orgasm at a greater speed.

And if she senses that her partner is going to take a long time to come and she feels her own orgasm approaching, she can increase his arousal first by using her hands and mouth on his penis before taking one of the woman-on-top positions in which she is better able to control the pace.

DOES IT MATTER?

Simultaneous orgasm is not the be-all and end-all of love-making and the loving couple recognize this. For matter, on some occasions, the quality of the other's orgasm is of greater importance than their own. And the wise lover recognizes always that by increasing the pleasure of their partner's orgasm, they greatly improve the quality of their own – if not on this particular occasion, then in the future.

Equally, there are occasions when it is not desirable for one partner to have an orgasm. If the woman is performing oral sex on the man, the advanced lover makes it clear that the quality of his climax is her only concern and it should be implicitly understood that he need not worry about her pleasure – at least not on this occasion.

And if, say, the man is using a vibrator on his partner before bringing her to orgasm manually or orally, she should be made to understand that there is no pressure on her to reciprocate.

DURING INTERCOURSE

Yet, no lovemaking session should be entered into with one, or both, partners feeling that simultaneous orgasm has to be the end result of their lovemaking. Apart from the fact that this is too clinical an approach to sex, it is also unrealistic. The way to approach any lovemaking session is to see simultaneous orgasm as a bonus and to concentrate on giving the other pleasure. In that way, the quality of orgasms – for both partners – will be increased and the lovemaking session will be what it should always be – a shared experience between two lovers.

And if one partner does not reach orgasm, it need not matter. There is always another time. One of the virtues of sex is that it can be practised at any time, as often as a couple like and – within reason – anywhere.

MALE LEAD

When two people arrange to make two things happen at the same time, one person generally has to compensate for the other in some way. And nowhere is this more true than in a couple's lovemaking. If arousal for the woman takes time, then the man will have to compensate by delaying his own climax and increasing the pace of her arousal. Alternatively, the woman can take the initiative and slow down the pace of the man. And if she is approaching climax without any signs of his, she will have to delay her own responses and speed up his.

THE MAN IN CONTROL

To speed up a woman's responses to your caresses, the quality of foreplay has to be what she likes best. And if you are already highly aroused you are going to have to hold back your own orgasm to help your partner achieve her's. Using words, kisses and caresses – and choosing a position where you are in control – should all help to hurry things up for her.

COME FIRST

If you have difficulty holding back your own orgasm, a good idea is to have one first yourself. This is because your second orgasm always takes longer. Only you will

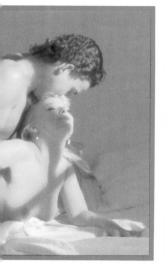

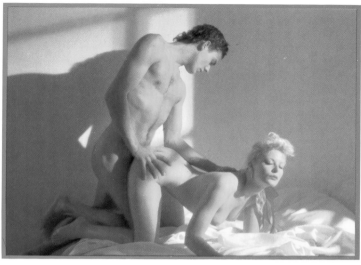

(left) As both your orgasms approach, you can increase the depth of penetration and stimulate her G-spot if your partner raises herself up on all fours

Skilful use of a dildo will soon increase your partner's level of arousal – use your other hand and your lips to caress her and encourage her to caress and kiss you as you bring her to the point of orgasm

Through masturbation, women are well aware of how to increase their own arousal levels. Use your hands and lips on your partner's body as she stimulates her clitoris or vulval area to bring herself closer to orgasm

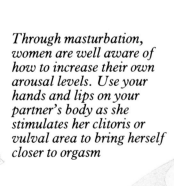

partner to bring you to orgasm – with her hands or mouth first. In an understanding relationship, your partner is going to be only too delighted to give you two climaxes in one lovemaking session, if the quality of her own climax is to be improved.

MAKE THE FOREPLAY GOOD

The choice of positions that you finally use to make love is important but, as in all lovemaking encounters – excluding quickie sex which has a charm of its own – the quality of the foreplay you choose to arouse your partner is crucial.

Make massaging her memorable and then kiss her

know if this is a wise course of action. Obviously, if it is going to leave you temporarily impotent for any great length of time it is not a realistic option. But, if you feel confident that you will be ready to have another orgasm within a reasonable time, ask your

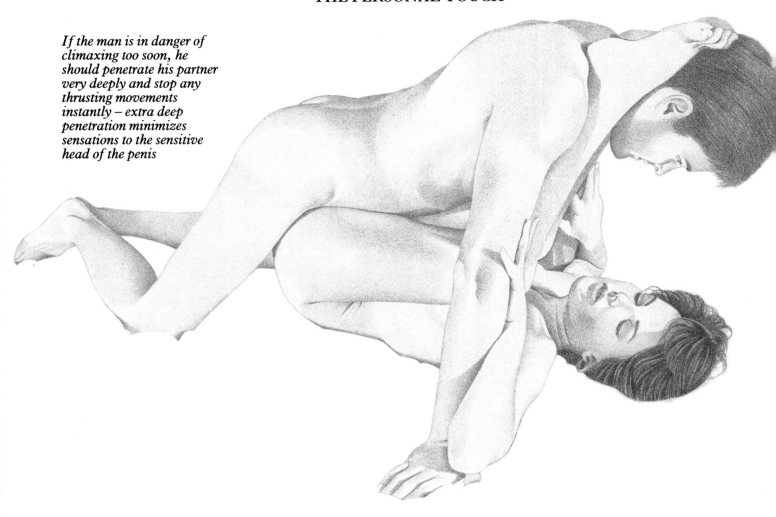

If the man is in danger of climaxing too soon, he should penetrate his partner very deeply and stop any thrusting movements instantly – extra deep penetration minimizes sensations to the sensitive head of the penis

all over. Use your fingers and tongue as creatively as you know how and in a way you know will bring her to the brink of orgasm. Talk to her, telling her what you want to do to her, telling her how desirable she is and how much you want her. If she likes you to use anglo-saxon words as you make love – then do so. Gauge from her reactions when to enter her.

CREATIVE USE OF THE VIBRATOR

If you have a vibrator or dildo, use that to bring her all the way to the brink of orgasm. Use it creatively over her body but pay special attention to her vulval area. Alternatively, get her to use it on herself and use your hands and lips to please her elsewhere. This way, the sensations are greatly multiplied.

You can caress either her back or front then use your fingers on her vaginal lips. Let her use the vibtrator in the way she likes best. If she uses it on her clitoris, use your fingers inside her vagina, varying the pace of the thrusting movements you use. If she prefers to insert the vibrator inside herself, then use your fingers or your tongue on her clitoris. When she has reached the brink of orgasm, then is the time to enter her. It is up to both partners to help regulate each other's orgasm.

ENCOURAGE FANTASY

If she likes to fantasize, encourage her to do so. There is no reason why she should not envisage whatever scene she wishes as you make love and this can easily be an important part of relaxing loveplay. And for many women, this is a classical way to bring them closer to orgasm as they let their mind roam free.

GET HER TO MASTURBATE

Because a woman knows her own sexual needs better than anyone – including her lover – it may make sense for you to encourage her to masturbate. This need not reduce you to the role of spectator, however – rather you should involve yourself in her pleasure. Kiss her lips, breasts, thighs, anus or whatever she likes as she brings herself closer to climax. Then, she can tell you when to penetrate her.

POSITIONS

Choose a position where you are in control and where you can stimulate her clitoris easily. The choice is yours, but it is best not to go for one of the more athletic positions where you need to concentrate on your own technique rather than your partner's needs. It is probably best to keep things simple.

☐ **Use the missionary position** Not without reason is this a position that a couple find that they return to time and again. It is both romantic – lovers can gaze at each other which in itself is highly arousing – and it is particularly suitable for a couple who are trying to coincide their orgasms, as they can gauge the other's reactions to what they are doing and see when they are other is approaching orgasm. Lie your partner back and open her legs as wide as possible and enter her. She may prefer to wrap her legs around your waist or perhaps put them over your shoulders so that you can go for deeper penetration. Allow her to choose which variation she prefers. Start thrusting slowly and encourage her to stimulate her clitoris as you concentrate on timing your orgasm with hers. Watch her and be guided by her reactions as to whether you should increase the pace and at what time. As her orgasm approaches, now is the time to throw caution and restraint to the winds and thrust as hard as possible. Lower your head and suck her breasts and kiss her lips as you both move towards orgasm.

☐ **Try a side entry position** Probably the most advantageous position in terms of versatility and ease of access – the man can easily stimulate his partner's clitoris as he makes love to her – is one where the man lies at right angles to his partner's body under her raised and parted thighs. Normally used as one of the more restful positions, there are no reason why it cannot be used more energetically. The woman is free to caress her clitoris or you can do it for her. It also gives the woman freedom of movement to turn her head towards you so that you can kiss and caress her and see when her orgasm is imminent. When you have entered her, kiss her breasts and body, always being guided by her needs as to how hard you should thrust. Also, from here, you can use your hands to stimulate her buttocks and anus if she likes.

☐ **Enter her from behind** If she has a sensitive G spot, a rear entry position is called for where you are thrusting towards the front wall of her vagina. The only disadvantage of this position for simultaneous orgasm is that access to her clitoris for the man tends to be limited. This is easily overcome, however, if the women stimulates herself. Get her to lie on her front, make sure that she is comfortable and get her to raise her buttocks as high as she can, so that she is literally offering herself up to you. Use your fingers to part her vaginal lips and enter her – she should be highly aroused and providing her own lubrication. If she is not, use saliva on her vulva. Encourage her to stimulate her clitoris and thrust slowly at first aiming for her G spot and concentrating on holding back your own orgasm. As the moment approaches, and if she likes this, you can use a finger to tease her anus and perhaps pop it in at the moment of orgasm.

MOVEMENT

In all these positions, many men concentrate almost exclusively on thrusting. But the creative lover can use his penis in other ways during intercourse – and in any position. Sadly, sideways movement of the penis is often ignored which is a pity because it has the twin advantages of feeling slightly less arousing to the man, thus giving him more control, and being highly stimulating for the woman.

So, when your penis is inside her vagina, resist the temptation to thrust as deeply as possible all the time and concentrate instead on sideways control. Move your hips and buttocks and try to hit the side walls of your partner's vagina. Then try rotating your penis inside her almost as if you were trying to stir round and around. Be inventive and experiment.

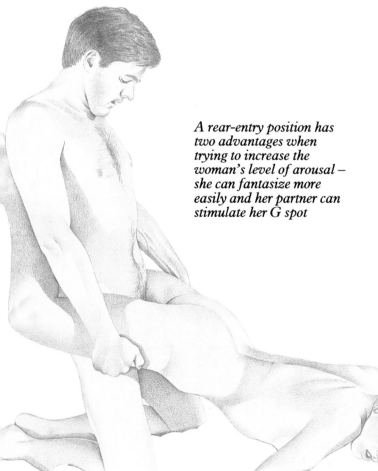

A rear-entry position has two advantages when trying to increase the woman's level of arousal – she can fantasize more easily and her partner can stimulate her G spot

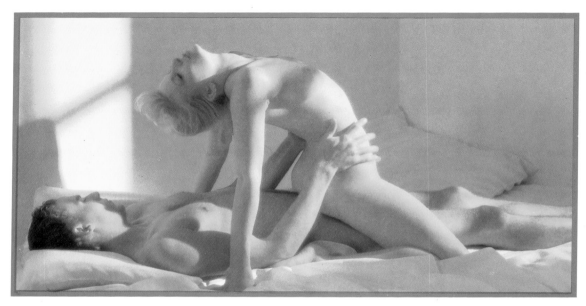

FEMALE LEAD

Probably the best way to slow down a man and delay his orgasm is to give him an earlier orgasm – before the main event – and then to use a woman-on-top position where you are in control. For many women, it can be important, as well as arousing, to dictate the pace at which lovemaking takes place.

GIVE HIM AN EARLIER ORGASM
Unlike in most creative foreplay where the aim is to give the other the most explosive orgasm possible, on this occasion it is a good idea to keep the pace of his earlier orgasm down. The reason for this is that if his orgasm is only an appetizer for the main event, it makes sense not to attempt to give him the most powerful ejaculation possible where all he may want to do afterward is relax or go to sleep.

USE A WOMAN-ON-TOP POSITION
There are a number of woman-on-top positions that the creative couple can use, but most of them come down to variations on two basic ones – with you facing towards your lover, or facing away from him.

☐ **Facing him** In the same way that the missionary position gives the man complete freedom to use his hands to explore your body and see you so that he can gauge your reactions, so too does this position. It also enables you to set the pace – speeding yourself up, perhaps by caressing your clitoris – and controlling the depth and frequency of his thrusting. It also allows you to use your body creatively – up and down and sideways as well as using a kind of grinding motion. Lay your partner down on his back, squat over his penis and use your hands to help him penetrate you as you ease yourself down on him.

Start off by using slow, short strokes, perhaps allowing only the top of his penis inside you and then,

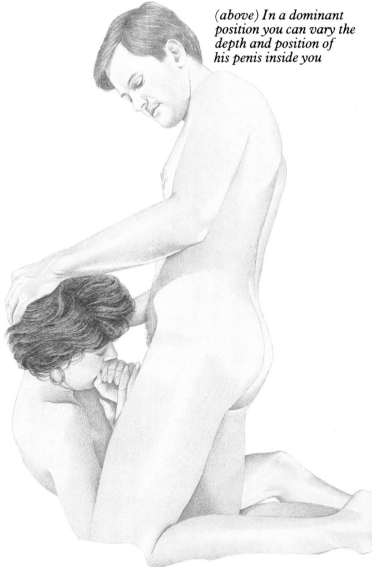

(above) In a dominant position you can vary the depth and position of his penis inside you

without increasing the pace, lengthen the strokes so that the whole penis is inside you. You can vary the depth of penetration by arching your back away from him or leaning over towards him. If his orgasm is approaching, you can suddenly start moving from side to side so that the friction against his penis is less.

Also, research has shown, perhaps surprisingly, that the deeper the penetration, the less arousing it is for the man. So, if he looks as if he is going to come too quickly lean forwards towards him, allowing him inside you as deeply as possible.

☐ **Facing away from him** This position has all the advantages of the other woman-on-top positions save one – you are unable to see your partner's reaction to what you are doing. This can be compensated for, however, by getting him to tell you if his own orgasm is close, or he can use a prearranged signal – perhaps tapping your back. You are allowed the same freedom of movement, however, as well as the bonus of being able to fantasize by looking away from him. Also, you can use your lover's penis in a more unhibited way. It can also be used as a starting-off position – the sight of

your buttocks may be particularly arousing for your partner – and as climax nears, you can turn around, keeping your partner's penis inside you. But be careful. Some men find that this movement immediately triggers off their climax.

SPEEDING UP THE MAN
If your partner takes more time than you do to reach orgasm then you need to place more emphasis on foreplay. Creative use of oral sex should bring him to the peak of orgasm and then you can use your body to control the pace of both your orgasms – this time to speed him up. And if you want a new bout of lovemaking your lips should serve to rearouse all but the most reluctant of men.

IF IT DOES NOT HAPPEN
Humans being what they are, simultaneous orgasm is not going to happen every time. But this need not matter. A couple who use any creative method to

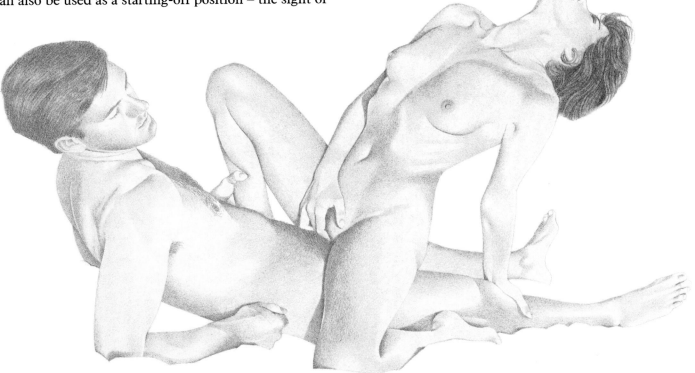

(left) If the woman is highly aroused and is approaching orgasm before her man, she should turn all her attention on to him; using her mouth and hands on his penis will soon increase his level of arousal and bring him closer to orgasm

This woman-on-top position has two advantages for the couple who are trying to synchronize their orgasms – they can see to gauge each other's level of arousal and the woman can stimulate herself easily

increase the quality of their loveplay should be happy with the extra rewards that it brings. If either partner comes afterwards, or fails to come during the session, the advanced lover will not feel disappointed. He or she will use their mouth, lips or body in some way to bring the other to orgasm or will accept that it can always happen another time. For if the sensual pleasure of both partners is increased, then simultaneous orgasm is a bonus – a delightful one admittedly – but no more than that.

ORAL SEX

Within a loving relationship, oral sex can be an integral part of a couple's sexual repertoire, and most find it a delightful and highly arousing form of lovemaking

FOR HER

A man's mouth can be highly erotic and arousing when used in the right way on almost any part of a woman's body. In reality, oral sex includes kissing and sucking of any part of her body – unfortunately most people concentrate on the genitals to the exclusion of other oral pleasures.

Almost all woman enjoy oral sex that does not involve the genitals. They see it as romantic as it shows how much their man loves them. When it comes to having their genitals kissed, licked and sucked things are rather different. Some women see this as the most intimate thing a man can do to, and for, them and so greatly value it as a sign of his total love. Others have been conditioned to think of their genitals as dirty and naughty and they cannot imagine anyone liking them, let alone wanting to kiss them.

At least some of these women can be persuaded to change their minds if, once they are aroused by clitoral or other stimulation, the man gently but firmly starts to kiss first around the vulva area and then the clitoris. Be careful not to tickle and make every effort to reproduce with your tongue what your partner usually does herself during masturbation and you will soon overcome the inhibitions.

NON-GENITAL ORAL SEX

Lie alongside your partner face to face. Kiss her face gently all over, not forgetting to suck her ear lobes, if she likes it. Kiss her mouth, lips and tongue and arouse her further by caressing her body with your hands. The beauty of almost all the oral sex positions is that they leave the hands free to caress and arouse other parts of the woman's body.

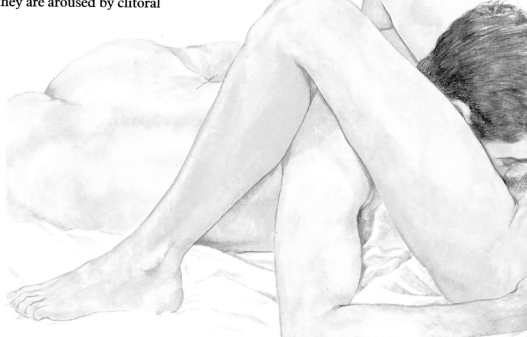

TIPS FOR ORAL SEX

☐ Clean your teeth.
☐ Shave.
☐ Agree with your partner that you are going to caress her in this way. This gives her a chance to:
☐ Trim her pubic hair or even shave the area.
☐ Wash her vulva, perineal and anal areas thoroughly.
☐ Leave off her panties or wear open-crotch panties so that you will be able to get down to things easily.
☐ Put in a fresh tampon and push the string inside if she is having a period.

Move down her body so that your head is on a level with her stomach. From here you can kiss her breasts, suck her nipples, put the whole of a breast into your mouth or blow on her nipples.

Run your tongue around her nipples and probe deeply with it into her breasts under the nipple and areola. Never bite, except very gently, and then not as she climaxes as you could do damage because she will be less sensitive to pain then.

This will all be especially arousing to the breast-centred woman. It is also a particularly good position for using during a period or in pregnancy. Some women have an orgasm when this much time and care are taken to fully arouse their breasts.

TRAVEL DOWNWARDS

Now move your mouth down onto her stomch. Lick and kiss her navel and run your mouth and lips all over her stomach, round and round in circles. Work down towards her vulva but, at this stage, do not touch it with either your hands or your mouth.

Lie in between your partner's feet, perhaps kneeling on the floor at the end of the bed. You can now kiss and suck her toes and feet. Some women so enjoy this that they nearly have a climax, even if the rest of the body is not touched. This is a good position for the woman who likes to caress her own breasts and/or clitoris while her partner caresses her feet orally.

Do not forget her hands. Get into any position you find comfortable and take her hand in yours or lie it, back downwards, on to the bed. Run your tongue all over it and between the fingers and then suck her fingertips and kiss her palms. Caress her palms with your tongue.

VARIATIONS

Once your partner has been aroused by non-genital oral contact she will probably be very receptive to genital oral contact. This is the best time to try, but go gently if she has any qualms about oral sex.

☐ The best position is probably with the woman lying flat on her back with her legs apart. The man lies in between her legs so that he can easily lick, kiss and suck any part of her genitals. A major problem with this is neck-ache, so prevent this by putting a pillow two (depending on how saggy your bed is) under her hips. This will raise the vagina and bring it into a better, more accessible position.

This position is good for licking and kissing the clitoris but less so for putting the tongue in the vagina or caressing the perineum or anus.

☐ A good variation of this position is for the woman to lie in the same way, but for the man to turn around to face her feet. He now has his genitals over her face and she can suck and kiss his penis if that is what they both enjoy. If not, he can angle his body so that she does not have his genitals in her face.

By supporting himself on his elbows, he is able to kiss her vulva and clitoris very easily. The main precaution here is to be sure not to put too much weight on the woman's body. It should all be distributed on the man's knees and elbows.

In this position the man can reach under his partner's thighs, pull them apart, and can open the outer lips so as to give the best possible access for oral sex. The skilful man can even insert the fingers of one hand (or both) into the vagina while kissing the clitoris and the vulval area. This is also an excellent position for the couple who like to use a dildo or vibrator in the woman's vagina while she is being caressed orally. The man can watch it going in and out and the woman's hands are free to caress him and she can suck his penis if she wants to.

☐ The woman lies with her hips on the edge of the bed and her feet flat on the floor. The man kneels between her thighs and kisses and rubs her vulva and

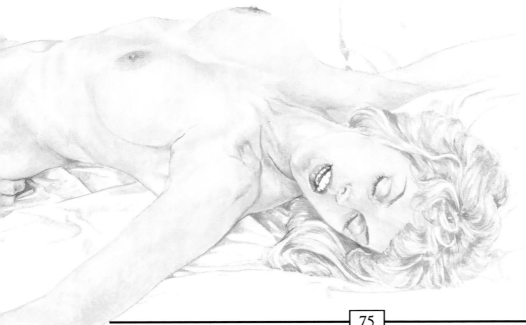

If the man places his hands under his partner's buttocks as she lies back on the bed, he can raise her body slightly to get her vulva at a level where he can kiss, suck or lick the whole area. However, this position allows little contact with other areas of the body

The woman supports her weight on her arms and her toes, aided by her partner who places one hand under her buttocks. Her partner is now ideally placed to caress her vulval area with his tongue

clitoris. As she becomes more excited the woman can pull her thighs back to her chest, but still keeping them apart so that he has access to her open vulva. This is an exceptionally good position for the woman who likes her man to insert his tongue into her vagina or to kiss her perineum.

All of this can be repeated with the woman lying on a table. This is in many ways more comfortable for the man because he has to bend down less as the woman's vulva is more level with his face.

☐ The man lies flat on his back and the woman kneels over his chest and gives him her vulva to kiss. She can, if she wishes, orally caress his penis. This position is good during pregnancy and allows the man to see her bottom, kiss her perineum and even to kiss her anus if they both want it. This position is best for the woman who likes such intimate lovemaking to be anonymous. She can face away from her partner's head and reach through between her open thighs to caress her clitoris as the man tongues her vagina.

☐ The man kneels down in front of the woman who stands, feet wide apart. He can now lick, kiss and suck her vulva underneath. This can be fun if the woman is fully dressed, apart from her panties. He is then covered by her skirt.

☐ As a variation of this, she can lean backwards on to something such as a high ledge or shelf – provided she can get herself into a comfortable position.

☐ Finally, for the adventurous couple, the man lies down on his back on the bed or the floor with his knees drawn up. The woman now kneels over his face, legs wide apart facing him, with her vulva over his mouth. She then leans backwards on to his knees and relaxes with her head over his knees. The vulva is exceptionally wide open and the man can push his tongue into her vagina and caress her vulva and clitoris with his mouth.

Her breasts are very exposed and can be played with or stimulated either by herself or the man. This is a somewhat tiring position but is fun for a change.

A relaxing position for the man, as he lies on his back on the bed while his partner kneels astride his face, leaning forward and supporting her weight on her arms. The man can caress her buttocks, open up her vulval area and pay close attention to her clitoris, vagina and perineum. Most women find this position highly arousing as they have the freedom to move their body

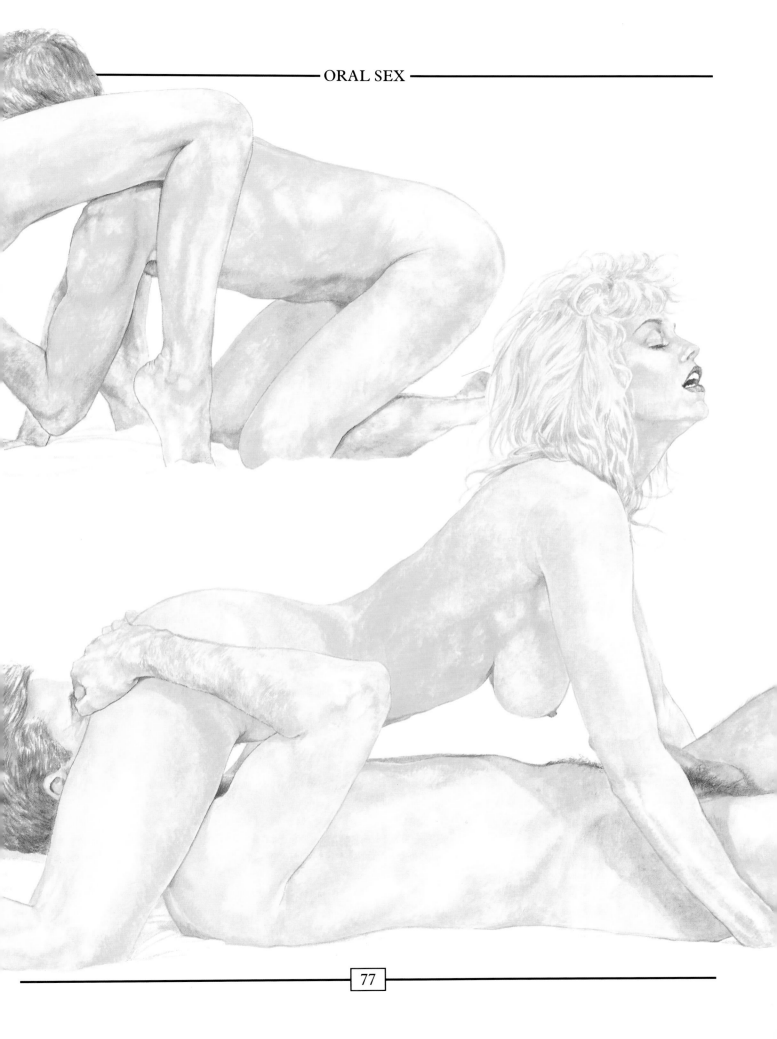

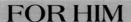

With the man lying on his back, his partner can control the action and caress him at the same time – a good position for the woman who is new to this type of lovemaking

FOR HIM

For the woman who likes to express her love in the most intimate way, oral sex will both delight and excite her partner on every occasion.

There are few men who are not flattered and highly aroused by their partner caressing their genitals orally. In a society in which so many women are still brought up to believe that they should not take an active part in sex, the sight and experience of a woman taking the initiative and pleasing her partner in this highly personal way is very exciting for most men.

There are many positions that are suitable and comfortable for fellating a man and any inventive couple will find those that suit and excite them best. It is useful to bear in mind when thinking about many oral sex positions that a couple's size is a consideration. A couple of near equal height will be able to achieve almost any of the positions described, but if the woman is more than six inches shorter than the man they will need to experiment to find the ideal position for them.

Before a woman fellates her partner, the couple should lay down some basic ground rules for performing oral sex.

☐ Any man who expects his partner to fellate him should always keep his penis and whole genital area scrupulously clean, especially under the foreskin.

☐ It is good manners to agree before any given episode including oral sex whether it is to be a part of foreplay or if it is to end in oral intercourse with the man ejaculating in the woman's mouth. Many couples have pre-agreed ideas on this, but for the couple who enjoy either, depending on the mood of the occasion, a secret sign understood only by them and without the needs for words, is usually all that is required. If you know that your man particularly wants to ejaculate in your mouth and you do not like swallowing semen, arrange to have a box of tissues handy so that you are able to discreetly spit it out.

☐ Whatever position you eventually go for, be sure that you are comfortable, and will not get tired easily. Most men tend to come very quickly with oral caresses but many couples like to spin things out, to tease the

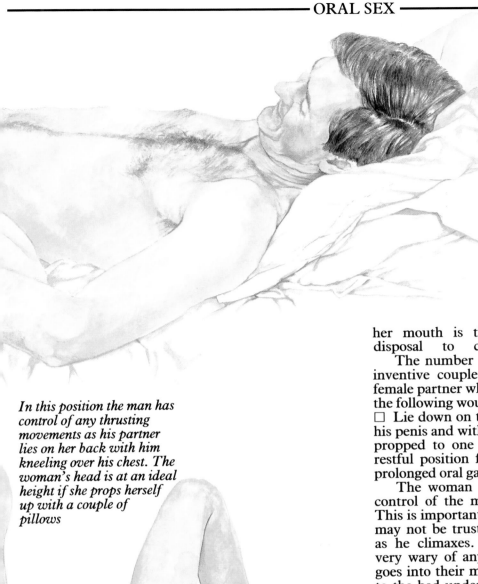

In this position the man has control of any thrusting movements as his partner lies on her back with him kneeling over his chest. The woman's head is at an ideal height if she props herself up with a couple of pillows

man by exciting him and then letting him go down for a while only to repeat the cycle. Any prolonged oral lovemaking like this calls for both parties to be comfortable and relaxed.

☐ Keep your teeth out of the way at all times.

☐ Keep your hands busy elsewhere so that he has the best possible stimulation – and not just to his penis.

VARIATIONS

Oral sex can be a prelude to genital intercourse, or a form of lovemaking on its own. And for the woman who wants to arouse her man again after a sex session,

her mouth is the most powerful weapon at her disposal to caress and excite him again.

The number of positions that can be used by the inventive couple is vast, but for the inexperienced female partner who is unfamiliar with oral sex, some of the following would make a good starting point.

☐ Lie down on the bed with your head at the level of his penis and with him on his back facing you, slightly propped to one side, with a pillow or two. This a restful position for both partners and is suitable for prolonged oral games.

The woman is on top of the penis and so is in control of the movement and depth of penetration. This is important for anyone fellating a new lover who may not be trusted to control the depth of thrusting as he climaxes. Some women are, understandably, very wary of any position in which the man's penis goes into their mouth with him on top. She is pinned to the bed under his body and can easily choke if he thrusts too deeply. Not only is this bad manners but it is also dangerous, as at the height of orgasm it is difficult for some men to control their actions and stop instantly if their partner is in danger of choking.

This position is also good for the woman who intends to fellate her man but not let him ejaculate in her mouth. She sucks and kisses him until she feels he is about to ejaculate and then by moving her head away, can let him ejaculate over her breasts, or even on to a paper tissue.

☐ Given that the penis likes to be pointing upwards, a very pleasant position is for the woman to lie with her head on the man's stomach and then to take the penis into her mouth. He can caress almost all of her body, can certainly reach down to touch her bottom and possibly her clitoris and the whole position is very restful and romantic. If she does not want to swallow the semen she can simply remove her head and continue to stimulate him manually until he ejaculates over his stomach.

☐ If the woman kneels over the man's body, facing

away from him, she can suck him while pressing her breasts and stomach against his stomach and chest. This position gives him a view of her bottom, anus, and vulva and this in itself can add to the excitement if he does nothing other than lie there with his eyes open and caress her body all over.

For the 'bottom-centred' man this is a very enjoyable position, as it is for the woman who enjoys displaying herself so openly.

☐ The woman can lie down on her front between the man's legs, raising herself on her elbows. She fellates her man from below. There is a danger in this position that the man's penis could be bent down towards his knees and be uncomfortable for him, so be careful. Almost all of her body, except her head, is out of his reach, so he cannot caress her much in this position. She does, however, face him and if he likes to watch his penis going in and out of her mouth he can prop his head up on a pillow. Her arms fix her in one position, strictly limiting what she can do with her hands, but she can caress his testes easily.

☐ The man kneels over the woman's chest facing her head and she takes his penis into her mouth. This is very restful for the woman but the man has to remain upright, which can be tiring over a long time. The woman is pinned down and cannot control the depth and rate of thrusting, which makes this a position suitable only for couples who know and trust each other very well.

If the woman does not want to swallow the semen she can find spitting it out very difficult in this position. But if she withdraws the penis before his climax she can then masturbate him to orgasm so that he ejaculates on to her chest. This simply entails him leaning backwards a bit or maybe even shifting his knees back.

In this position, the woman can reach around to fondle and knead his bottom and she can also easily caress and stroke his stomach and thighs.

☐ The man kneels up on the bed or the floor with his body upright. The woman lies flat on her back in front of him with her head under his genitals. She can now suck his penis as it hangs downwards. Movement is not very good for either partner but it leaves the woman's hands free to caress her breasts and clitoris and he can easily ejaculate over her chest if she does not want him to come into her mouth.

☐ The man stands and the woman kneels in front of him and takes his penis into her mouth. She can now control the speed and depth of penetration to exactly what she likes. If she senses he is about to climax, she can pull her head away if she does not want semen in her mouth. He will then be able to ejaculate on to her breasts, over the rest of her body, or into a tissue.

This is also a good postion for the woman who likes a dildo or vibrator inside her while she fellates her partner. She inserts the dildo and sits on it trapping it between her feet. She can now move up and down on the dildo while fellating her man. If she wants, she can reach down and caress her clitoris at the same time.

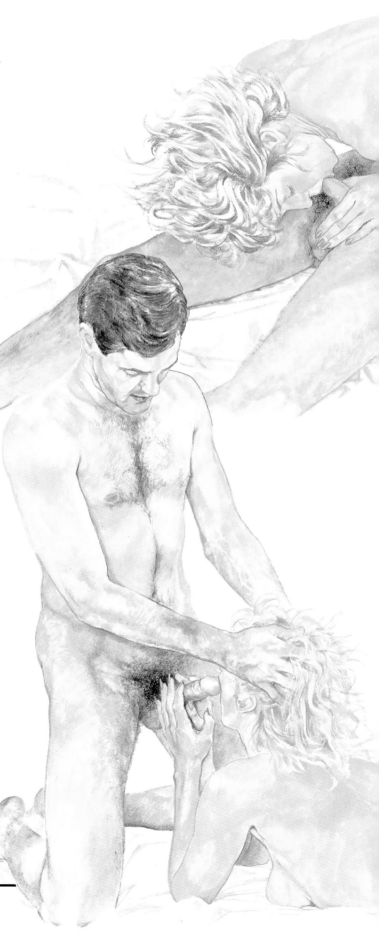

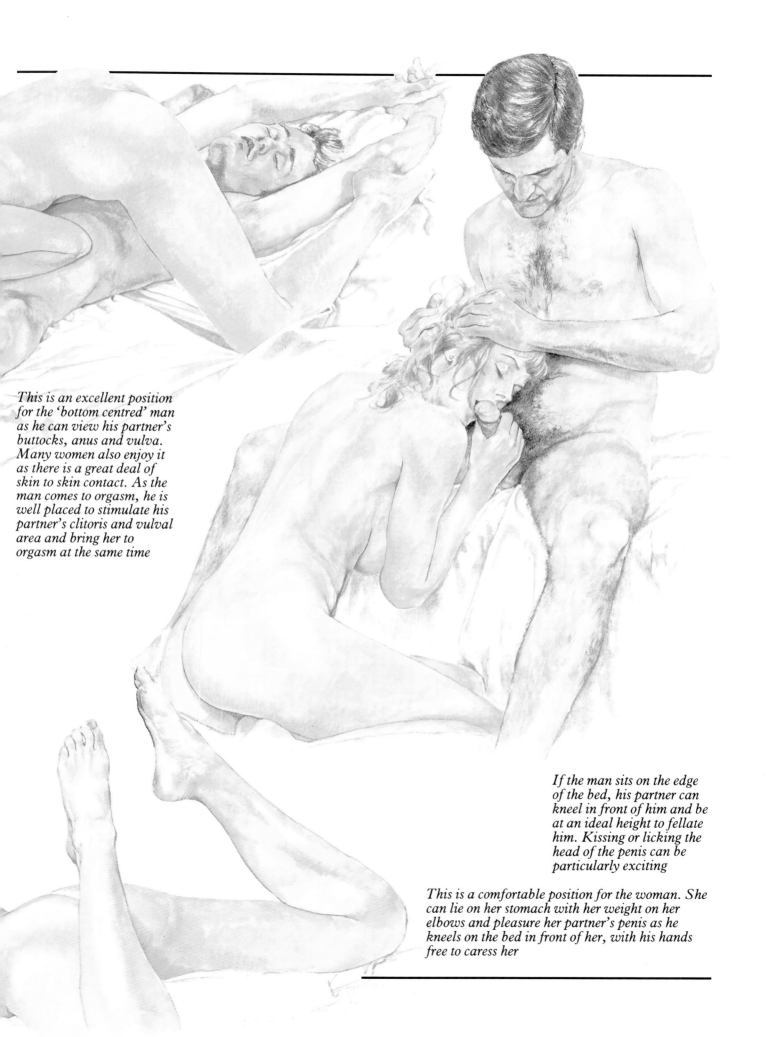

This is an excellent position for the 'bottom centred' man as he can view his partner's buttocks, anus and vulva. Many women also enjoy it as there is a great deal of skin to skin contact. As the man comes to orgasm, he is well placed to stimulate his partner's clitoris and vulval area and bring her to orgasm at the same time

If the man sits on the edge of the bed, his partner can kneel in front of him and be at an ideal height to fellate him. Kissing or licking the head of the penis can be particularly exciting

This is a comfortable position for the woman. She can lie on her stomach with her weight on her elbows and pleasure her partner's penis as he kneels on the bed in front of her, with his hands free to caress her

IMAGINATIVE SEX

Once the first flush of love has faded, a little imagination can keep the momentum going

By the time most couples have been together for a few months, and certainly after several years, they usually know each other's personality and desires quite well and are settled into a sexual routine that they find they can cope with. Studies suggest that most couples have the minimum of sexual activity they can get away with once the first flush of enthusiasm wears off. This comes about as both partners adjust to each other's needs.

Some couples have sex with almost clockwork regularity, while others wait for a familiar signal – like putting on a certain kind of clothing or kissing 'good-night' in a particular way. All too often, this routine approach leads to routine sex – safe, predictable, boring lovemaking. As a result, many couples do not experiment at all in their sex lives after a set stage.

TAKING SEX FOR GRANTED

Closely linked to all this is the feeling – unconscious in most people's minds – that once you are married you can somehow stop making an effort and your partner will just have to accept it. Many of the couples who go to sexual and marital counselling complain that things used to be fine, but that one, or both, now take the other for granted sexually, give little, make few demands in return and so feel bored. This is too easily leads to a search for sex outside the relationship, and things begin to go badly wrong.

Many of us fall into a sexual rut because we fear that what we imagine would be good to try would be unacceptable to our partner. To suggest something which sounds perverted or odd exposes us to being rejected, even ridiculed. And a number of couples say they fear that suggesting something unusual might put their partner off them for a while – so depriving them of such sex as they already have.

It is probably fair to say that most women still see sex as something that is done to them, although this is less applicable to younger women. In general, however, most women in our culture look to the man to come up with the ideas. But the simple truth is that many men just do not have any creative ideas – and, of those that do, many unconsciously see their partner as too 'pure' or 'nice' to want to indulge in them, and so leave them unmentioned.

This notion is the result of many repeated child-

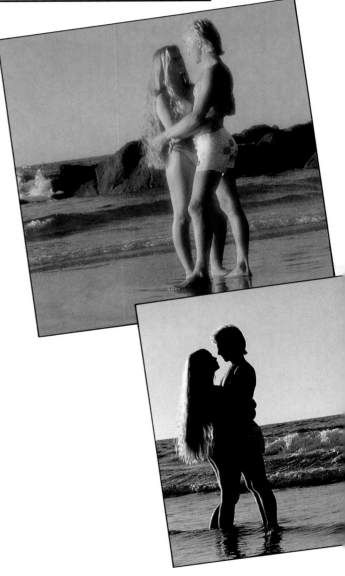

WHAT COULD BE MORE ROMANTIC THAN AN EMPTY BEACH AS THE LIGHT FADES?

Few people can resist the sensuality of the beach – the sun, sand and surf. The truly imaginative couple can have a holiday romance every year – with each other

hood messages that are transmitted unconsciously from parents to their children. A young man can be especially liable to be affected by this when his young (previously mistress-like) wife has a baby. She now becomes, in his unconscious mind, a sacred Madonna and, like his own mother, sexually unavailable. It is no coincidence that many affairs among young couples occur around pregnancy and birth – especially around the time of the first birth.

So, many men will not – or perhaps cannot – see their partner as an earthy female with real sexual needs and, because of the way some girls are brought up in our culture, they do not go out of their way to express their sexual desires. To do that could label them as tarty or cheap.

BREAKING THE MOULD

The problem is how to break out of this mould without causing havoc within the relationship – how to relieve the boredom without jeopardizing the good things. Most of us enjoy certain aspects of the predictability of a loving relationship, partly because it is comfortable, partly because it does not need working at in a demanding world in which we are so often striving and coping with change. Experimentation can have its price for some because it causes concern in an area of life in which they were safe and secure.

Yet the joys to be found in being more imaginative can far outweigh such disadvantages, especially in a

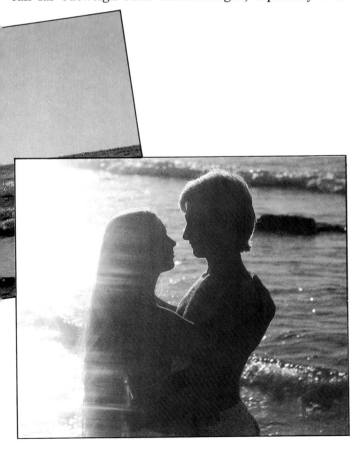

couple who are sensitive to each other's anxieties and know how to cope with them.

Breaking established routines can add excitement to life and stolen moments can be exhilarating. Spontaneous sex can prove that couples still find each other attractive, and are not simply responding to being turned on at prescribed times. The whole relationship can become more open, more honest, more relaxed, with couples talking about sex in a way they had not thought possible before.

Used properly and wisely, imaginative sex games will not endanger an existing and enjoyable sex life, but can provide ways of enriching your current 'repertoire'.

The golden rule is to keep an open mind. What appears ridiculous – or even perverted – to one partner may just be the bit of fun the other might like.

USE YOUR IMAGINATION

Imagination in this context does not mean fantasy. A fantasy is a conscious, or unconscious, mental device that enhances or creates sexual arousal, but imagination is almost entirely a conscious faculty that we use to enhance any activity in our lives – not just sex.

Some people are much more imaginative than others, of course, and this has both benefits and disadvantages. On the positive side such individuals come up with great ideas for the home, the family, their sex life or their job. This can be fine up to a point, but can be very disruptive if it gets out of control. All imagination, except in the hands of the fiction writer, has to have at least some bounds if it is to be acted out in real life.

Living with someone who is highly imaginative can be a real chore as well as a pleasure, if only because what seems to satisfy everyone else appears to leave them restless and dissatisfied. This does not matter too much in most spheres of life because their needs can be met elsewhere – perhaps outside the home and certainly outside the relationship – but when it comes to sex, most of us are supposed to find the answers to all our needs at home.

'True love', sexually as well as emotionally, is supposed to last for a couple's lifetime.

This is, for all but the luckiest, a forlorn hope, yet by thinking and behaving more imaginatively about sex any couple can greatly enhance their lives together.

NO HIDING PLACE

For the majority of couples, the most popular place for making love is the bedroom – preferably just before they go to sleep. Yet surprisingly large numbers make love in the sitting-room, bathroom or shower, at any time of the day.

Semi-public places are, and always have been, a great attraction for the imaginative couple. The secrecy involved and the chance of being spied on, or caught, can add spice to the experience, rather than cause nervous failure. It goes without saying that you have to be careful not to offend people and be discreet

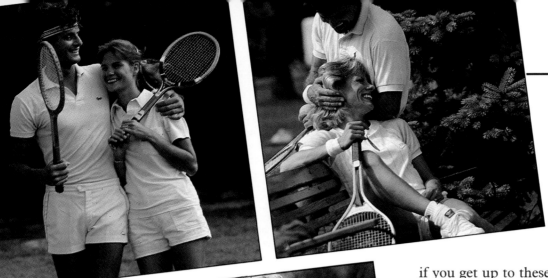

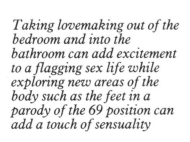

AFTER AN ENERGETIC GAME OF TENNIS, THERE ARE ALWAYS POSSIBILITIES

For the sporting couple, competitive sports generate a sense of exhileration and well-being, whether you win or lose. After a shower, what could be more natural than making love?

if you get up to these games, but making love in a car park or under the stars on the beach can be deliciously exciting – for a change.

Making love in cars has real disadvantages unless you are both very small or the car is very big. If you let your imagination run too wild you will end up with backache and neckache at best, and cramps and pulled muscles at worst. Do not have sex on the move. Some men greatly enjoy oral sex or being masturbated while they drive, but this is extremely dangerous since concentration levels fall dramatically after a certain point in the proceedings.

When people are on holiday they tend to be more adventurous than normal. They feel relaxed and, to some degree or other, they discard their normal roles. Some women only ever have an orgasm on holiday – when they think the children cannot hear them climaxing, for example – and others take on almost a different personality in a foreign place where they are quite unknown. This is why so many holiday romances work so well. It is as if time stands still and the individual can be someone else, if only for two weeks. Some long-standing couples have holiday romances with each other like this every year – you do not have to be single to enjoy them.

SPONTANEOUS SEX
At the heart of imaginative sex is, very often, the secret of spontaneity. Some couples are never spon-

Taking lovemaking out of the bedroom and into the bathroom can add excitement to a flagging sex life while exploring new areas of the body such as the feet in a parody of the 69 position can add a touch of sensuality

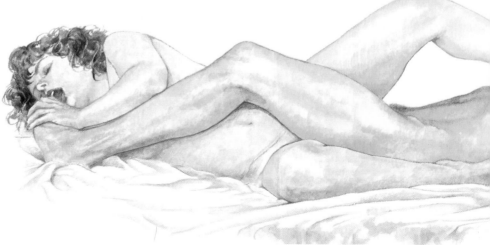

taneous and many make love on a fixed, regular basis, even on the same night of the week, each week. This may seem absurd to a more 'flexible' couple, but almost certainly fits in perfectly well with the rest of such couples' lives – predictable, routine, expected.

Yet for a large number of people 'quickie' sex is great. Indeed some women have orgasms only with quickie sex. They like to be taken hard and fast, with no questions asked. This proves to them that they are so desirable that their man cannot help himself wanting them, and this is highly flattering to their femaleness.

Instant sex can also be very pleasurable for the man both physically and psychologically, who, under other circumstances, might well have felt he had to work hard at producing an orgasm for his partner.

A number of men (whether they admit it or not) find the modern trend towards women's higher expectations in bed tedious, and long for the day when a woman was or seemed satisfied with a 'quick one'. Early in the morning is a good time for 'quickies', provided you do not have a partner who is too sleepy-headed in the morning.

BE PREPARED

Ironically, you have to be alert to the possibilities of, and be prepared for, spontaneous sex. This sounds like taking the fun away – but an unwanted baby is no fun either. Being contraceptively safe is a must – even the sexiest location and the most enjoyable 'quickie' can be blighted and doomed to failure if the woman is unsafe. Always take a sheath with you or even a diaphragm if you think 'spontaneous' sex is likely to occur and you are not on the Pill.

This is, of course, one of the major advantages of the Pill and sterilization – spontaneous sex becomes safe, and therefore easier, in every sense.

Once you are 'safe' you should think about the nature of your clothing. If you reckon that spontaneous sex with your man is on the cards leave your underwear off or wear open-crotch tights or knickers, and wear things that are easily removed. The tease of masses of small buttons or several layers of things may be fun in theory, but they are nothing but a nuisance in the heat of the moment. T-shirts that can be pulled up or off, bras that open in front, suspenders and stockings rather than tights – these are just a few ways of preparing yourself for sex in imaginative, spontaneous settings.

When thinking about planning for imaginative sex, do not aim for a seven course blow-out of a gourmet meal each time. Once you have agreed that, eventually, you will try most things, the occasions on which to indulge them will arise. Do not lose heart if your imaginative sex exploits turn out differently from how they were planned – there is always another day.

It is essential to point out that, while the 'quickie' has a special place in sex – and a charm all its own – it relies to a great degree for success on mutual physical knowledge. This knowledge – about what is physically possible for a partner, their and your rates of response, areas that excite and those that do not – can only be gained from longer lovemaking sessions.

In this sense the established couple have more chance of enjoyable spontaneous sex than the brief encounters of strangers in semi-pornographic movies.

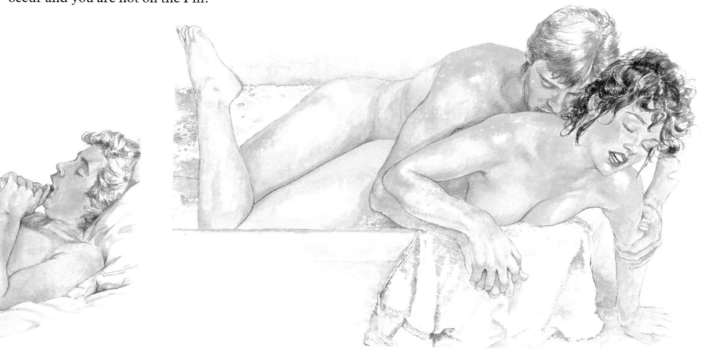

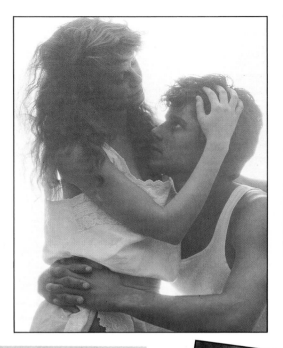

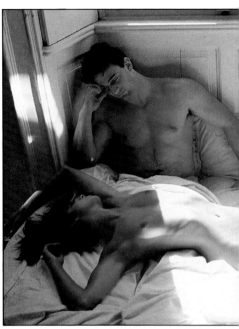

Making love, simply because you are in the mood, is just as important as being highly imaginative. Taking off your clothes and jumping into bed each night may be a natural trigger to lovemaking but you need not restrict sex to the midnight hour. If the mood takes you during the day, slowly undressing your partner can be incorporated...

IMAGINATION AND REALITY

Why don't we do it in the road? ran the Beatles' song. Well, that may be a little uncomfortable, not to mention dangerous to all concerned, and against the law. But there are more sensible venues which, simply by their very nature, add something to having sex. Even if a couple make love just as they do in the bedroom, it has to feel different on the beach at night, or in the garden.

SLEEP
During deep sleep, a woman's body relaxes profoundly and her vagina opens widely. A careful partner can lick his partner's vulva and even insert several fingers into her vagina without waking her. Some women sleep so deeply that they can be penetrated from behind, without stirring. A woman used to the feel of her lover's body round and in hers may well enjoy this in a state of semi-consciousness. Similarly, a woman who knows her partner's likes and dislikes may be able to do magical things to him during the night.

All this is not so ambitious or outrageous as it may sound. Many couples have different clocks and levels of tiredness, and this can be a way of compensating. But do not do it if your partner hates being woken.

WAKING UP
Sex on waking, or on the verge of waking, can be a wonderfully rewarding – and for some, very different – kind of feeling from 'evening sex'. Some women, especially, say they feel totally unable to resist and want to let themselves be taken over in the twilight time between sleeping and waking. Many men have

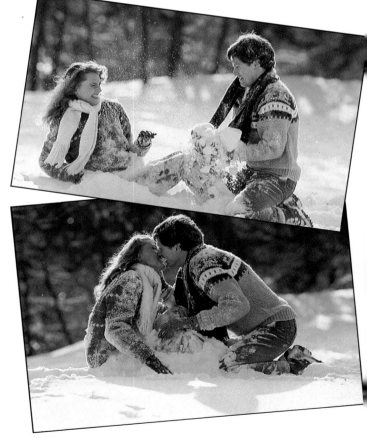

EVEN A COLD WINTER'S DAY CAN BE SEXY

The sharpness and fun of the snow can make a couple's thoughts turn to making love later – perhaps in front of a blazing log fire

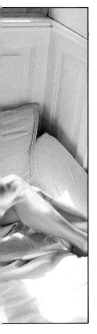
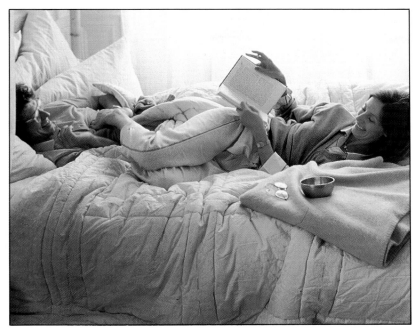

... into your lovemaking routine. In the middle of the afternoon, making love as the sun streams in can add a new openness to a relationship. And leisurely weekend mornings are also a favourite time for lovers. A lie-in with a good book, or the Sunday papers, can easily set the scene for a bout of lovemaking before deciding how to spend the rest of the day

erections on waking, and although there may be pressure to go to the toilet, sexual diversions can usually win.

A number of people are slow wakers, however, so do not be disappointed if you do not receive a riotous response from your partner at this time of day. Perhaps it is best to keep morning sex for weekends and holidays, when other demands and timetables are not so pressing.

Morning sex is almost impossible if you have children. Little ones wake up early and need changing and feeding, while bigger ones may be upset or not approve if they see or hear something. One answer for 'family' couples is to rearrange their sex lives – perhaps staying at a hotel or a friend's (empty) house or flat once in a while.

THE BATHROOM

The shower or bath is a natural venue for sex. For one thing, you are already undressed. Wash together or, maybe, make love together. It does not have to be that 'advanced' – simply soaping each other all over is a pleasant skin game – but intercourse in the bath is something a little different, even if the plumbing does get in the way. One word of warning soap can sting the urethra like it can sting the eyes.

Sex in the swimming pool has great possibilities because of the relative weightlessness involved. Some of those seemingly impossible positions featured on Hindu temples suddenly become attainable because the woman is now light enough to prop up. Needless to say, perhaps, this is a pastime for the private pool rather than the public baths.

The sea (after dark unless extremely private) is even better. The salt helps buoyancy and there is no chlorine as a potential irritant. Shoreline sex does have disadvantages; sand can be somewhat abrasive.

SPORT AND BONDAGE

Some couples are turned on by making love in a profusion of sweat after some energetic sport – squash, for example – and some women like the 'manly' smell of fresh sweat. The problem here, of course, unless you are extremely wealthy, is one of privacy.

Bondage can be a stimulating change to 'straight' sex. The idea is not to make your partner do something they would not do if they were not tied up – it is to enable you to tease them until they beg to be brought to orgasm. You have to agree on a set of ground rules, and always have a release signal which is obeyed without question, no matter how tempting the alternatives. Almost all women like to be overpowered sometimes, and most men have a need to be dominated, if only in a mild way and very occasionally. The possibilities are endless, from tied wrists to full-blown 'S and M'.

Care, however, must always be the watchword.

DRESSING UP

This can be a major factor in imaginative sex, since everybody harbours some kind of lust in terms of dress. It does not have to be a costume drama – a minimum of props can suffice with the right creative approach.

An ironic alternative is to make love with all your clothes on. All too often sex happens with nothing or merely nightclothes on, but doing it fully clothed is different and a natural consequence of spontaneous sex. All it needs is to take out the man's penis and push the woman's panties aside . . .

FOOD

Nearly everybody appreciates the sensuality of a candlelit meal for two lovers, but food can be a good deal more direct than that. Anything that needs handling to eat – asparagus, chicken legs, luscious fruits – can be extremely erotic to the watching man as the woman sucks them lingeringly before chewing and swallowing them.

But why not combine food with sexual activity? Put cream or ice-cream on the skin and lick it off – anything creamy is sexually symbolic. Lick something sticky off her nipples, or off his penis. The endless possibilities are left to your own imagination.

PHOTOGRAPHS

This really is a case of each to his or her own. More men than women are stimulated by visual pornography, but why not indulge in taking your own? Most commercial laboratories will process pinups and even mildly erotic material. For more explicit material use a polaroid camera.

MIRRORS

Many people get turned on by looking at themselves and/or their partner in mirrors. This creates an exciting voyeuristic element – but without having other people present. Either sex may be stimulated by seeing themselves masturbate or being tied up. Some lovers, it must be said, merely find them obtrusive.

LUBRICATION

The best lubricant for most areas of sex is saliva. It is always available and at the right temperature. But things can dry up, and anyway it can be fun experimenting with various harmless creams and jellies. A very wet vagina can be helpful to the man with premature ejaculation because it stimulates his penis less and he can last longer.

Some couples really enjoy shaving the woman's pubic hair, removing it with creams or foams, or even creating special shapes – like a heart.

PERIODS

It is quite possible to make love during a period. While some women suffer considerably during their periods, others actually feel sexy at that time, and can find it a turn-on because it can prove how much their man loves them.

If the tampon must remain in place, you can still have shallow, labial intercourse in the vulva.

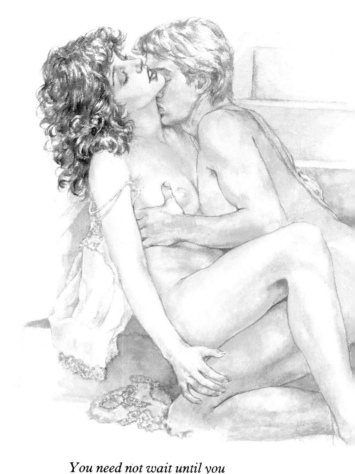

You need not wait until you reach the bedroom? Why not make love on the stairs, or add excitement by trying a new position?

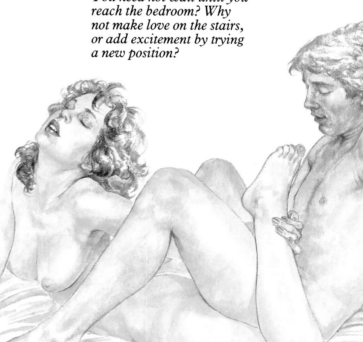

BIRTH CONTROL

Why not take steps to make contraception more of a turn-on instead of a turn-off?

Putting a sheath on a man, or inserting a diaphragm into a woman, can be a sexual adventure in itself. Almost anything, used imaginatively, can be incorporated into your love life and be more part of loveplay. Pleasure is, after all, intensely personal.

There are a few further suggestions that may help to make your lovemaking more imaginative and add spice to your sex life. Some may not appeal to either of you, but others may appeal to both. But if you try one or two, you may just find that your relationship with your partner is given a new boost – and then you can have fun experimenting.

It is a little like oysters or snails – how do you know you will not love them until you have tasted one?

REAR ENTRY

Although some people are put off by its animal symbolism and the lack of face-to-face contact, rear entry is tried by many couples and has a lot going for it – notably the possibility of deep penetration, ease of control, and the pushing of the pelvis against the buttocks.

An exciting variation is for the woman to kneel on the bed with her face down, her hands clasped behind her back. The man kneels behind and she hooks her legs over his and pulls him to her with them. He then puts a hand on each shoulder and gently pushes her down on to the bed. This position opens up the vagina as the man withdraws on each stroke – and pumps air into it when he thrusts. The combination of deep penetration and pumped air stretches the vagina a long way, often causing great pleasure but sometimes causing pain if it is taken too far. There is no danger that the air can do any harm because it can escape around the penis. The only disadvantage in this sense is that when the woman turns over she emits the 'wind' in an extremely noisy way.

Never, never, blow air into the vagina. It can kill.

BREASTS

While it is true that the sensitivity of women's breasts varies considerably, few couples make enough creative use of them in lovemaking, and most men literally pay them little more than lip service on their way to other areas. The imaginative woman will caress her partner all over with her breasts, and form a channel in which to caress the penis back and forth in a wonderfully sensual form of masturbation. And, when the man comes, why not massage the breasts with the semen?

SOME OTHER IDEAS

The armpit can make a surprisingly effective receiver for the penis, provided that the friction is on the shaft and not the glans (head). Opinions appear to vary on whether hair helps or not, but few women are likely to change such a basic personal habit because of occasional sex.

Feet can also be highly erotic – indeed some disciples of reflexology believe that, by rubbing a certain area of the foot firmly in an anticlockwise motion, it is possible to bring a person to orgasm. And just as the armpit can be used as a substitute vagina, so a big toe can be used as a substitute penis.

Start by covering your freshly washed foot in oil. You can then stimulate your partner's clitoris with your big toe before inserting it carefully into her vagina. Keep the toenails clipped.

Standing naked and exploring each other's bodies allows almost head-to-toe skin contact and can be an exciting prelude to sex. Also, eating can be a sensual experience if you are prepared to share – and not just fruit. Try smearing cream over your lover's body, then licking it off slowly

SEX AND MOVEMENT

Many couples limit the extent of their movement in intercourse. Yet there are positions which allow considerable scope for experiment with movement to improve the quality of their lovemaking

For most people, sexual release is impossible without some form of movement. A limited number of women can have an orgasm simply by thinking about something sexy, but the vast majority of men and women need to have their genitals stimulated before they reach a climax.

MOVEMENT AND MASTURBATION
Men, when masturbating, encircle the penis with most of their fingers and move the skin up and down rhythmically until orgasm. All other movement is secondary.

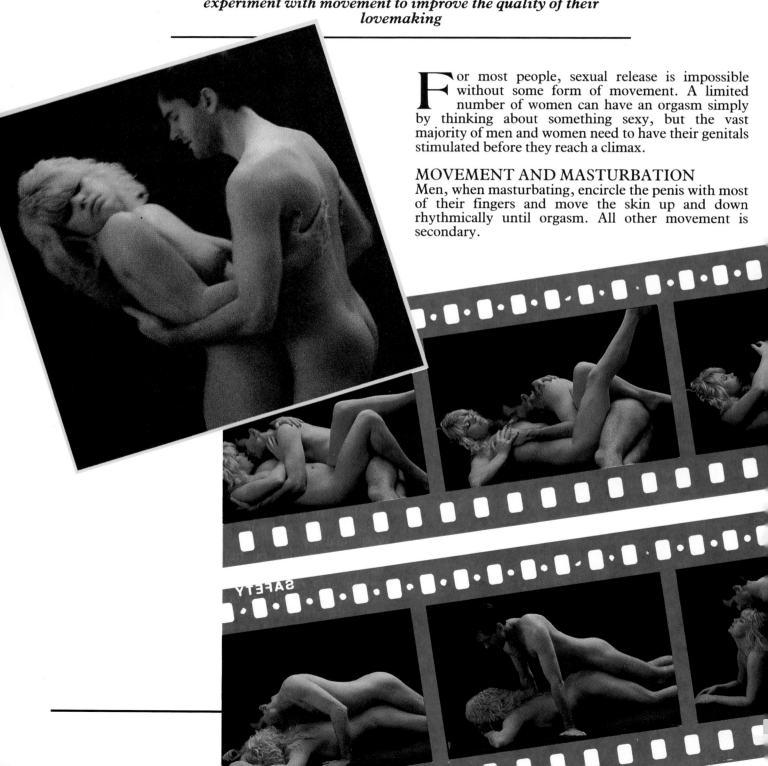

A woman masturbating is rather more complex, because although she usually needs to move the foreskin of her clitoris on its head (just as a man does with his penis), this can be done directly or indirectly. If done directly, it can be carried out using a finger, her man's tongue, or a vibrator. Each produces very different types of movement all of which, in turn, produce different sensations.

A finger can be made to move slowly or quickly, lightly or firmly, with very different stroke lengths and with very different pressures. Altering any one of these can make all the difference between success and failure to produce an orgasm. Often, women say that their partner-induced orgasms are sexier and more satisfying than those they gain themselves during masturbation.

A man's tongue can be used to stimulate both clitoris and vagina. Indeed, its movement over the whole vulval area can be extremely sensuous for many women. It is like no sensation she can produce herself.

Vibrators are all about movement. They produce a fine vibration that powerfully stimulates the clitoris and vulval area. This type of movement simply cannot be produced in any other way. Unfortunately, many women do not get the best out of their vibrators. The secret is to use fresh batteries or to have a main's-operated vibrator.

INDIRECT MOVEMENT
Usually, during intercourse the clitoris is stimulated indirectly as the penis is thrust in and out of the vagina. This movement pulls on the inner lips which are in turn attached to the hood of the clitoris. Physical in-and-out movement in the vagina therefore stimulates the head of the clitoris even though the penis is not touching it.

This is not always the case, however, and many women experience no clitoral stimulation at all from any amount of penis-in-vagina thrusting and need direct stimulation to be applied to the clitoral area.

MOVEMENT DURING INTERCOURSE
According to the gentry of Victorian times, 'ladies do not move'. A lady was supposed to be sexless, and

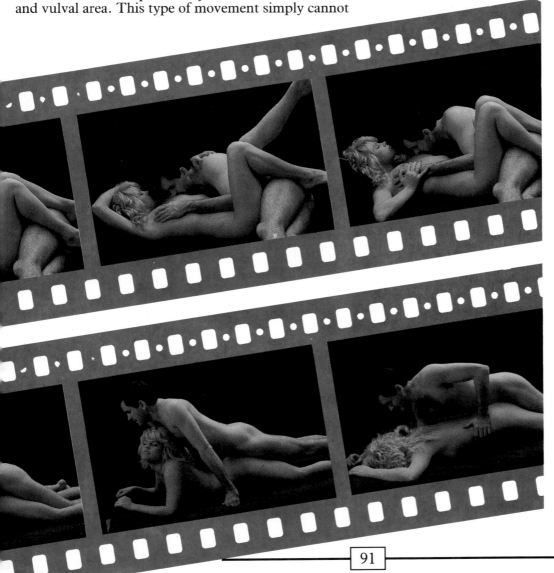

certainly would not be so crude as to move her body, just in case the man thought she was enjoying herself.

This is a harmful concept that is unfortunately still in existence. Clinical experience shows that some women, even now, lie beneath their partner with their legs open and remain motionless throughout the act of intercourse. To take a more active role would seem to them to be unacceptable 'tarty' and willing. Such sexually inhibited women believe that sex is something a man does to a woman, and that women are passive receptacles of men's lusty desires.

At the opposite end of the scale are men who have trouble controlling ejaculation. Such men can find highly active women difficult to cope with, because movement makes them come too soon. But an older man, or one with a tendency to slow ejaculation, will welcome his partner's active movements.

A woman can move in any position that leaves her body free enough to do so. Rear-entry positions are exceptionally good, because both partners are free to move for either pleasure or comfort.

MEN AND MOVEMENT

Men need to experience penile movement during intercourse, or they will not have an orgasm. They enjoy thrusting movements of various speeds and depths, but tend to thrust deeply as their orgasm becomes inevitable. For a man to obtain the most pleasure during intercourse, he usually tries to produce a situation in which the movements are as close as possible to those he uses during masturbation. This will, of course, differ from man to man. Some like long, slow movements and others short, jerky ones. These desires differ from time to time, and most people like to ring the changes, even during one lovemaking episode.

WOMEN AND MOVEMENT

Women have a wider range of pleasurable movements to enjoy. Thrusting is a favourite, but if a woman is on top she can thrust herself on to the penis (varying the depth of penetration to suit her and her man), or she can rotate her pelvis so that the penis is swept around the top of the vagina. The best way to imagine this is to pretend that the penis is a felt-tip pen inserted deeply into the vagina. The woman can now draw circles with the tip.

A woman can also contract the vaginal opening or her deep pelvic muscles. If she contracts her muscles as the penis moves inwards, and releases the pressure as it moves outwards, her man may very quickly be brought to orgasm.

Some women have learned to control their pelvic muscles to such a degree that they can produce an orgasm in a totally motionless penis by 'milking' it with these muscles. This is highly stimulating not only for their partners, but also for themselves.

The woman with a sensitive G spot can angle her body when in an on-top position to get her partner's penis tip right on the spot until she climaxes.

INTERCOURSE

The amount of movement each partner is capable of when making love depends very much on the position they have adopted. Some positions allow each partner to move freely, while others limit the movement of both partners, but allow for deeper penetration by the man.

Positions that allow full stroke movement:
☐ The woman kneels on a bed or low stool or lies over the edge of something higher (such as a table) and the man enters her from behind.
☐ The woman lies back in a deep chair with her legs apart. The man kneels in between her legs and penetrates her.
☐ The woman lies on her back with her knees up and her feet flat on the bed. The man supports his weight on his hands and penetrates her from above.
☐ Use the same position but the woman puts her ankles over his shoulders.
☐ The woman lies on her tummy with her hips on a pillow. The man approaches her from behind and, supporting himself on his hands, penetrates her.
Positions that allow full penetration, but little movement:
☐ The man sits on a simple chair. The woman faces away from him (or towards him) and sits on his penis.

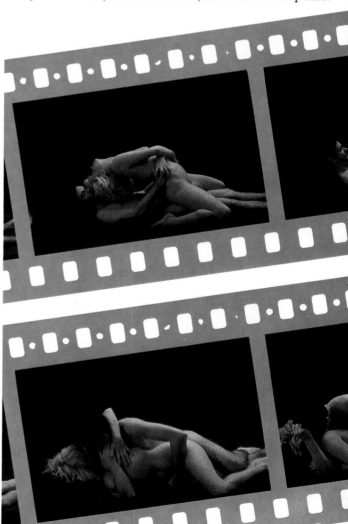

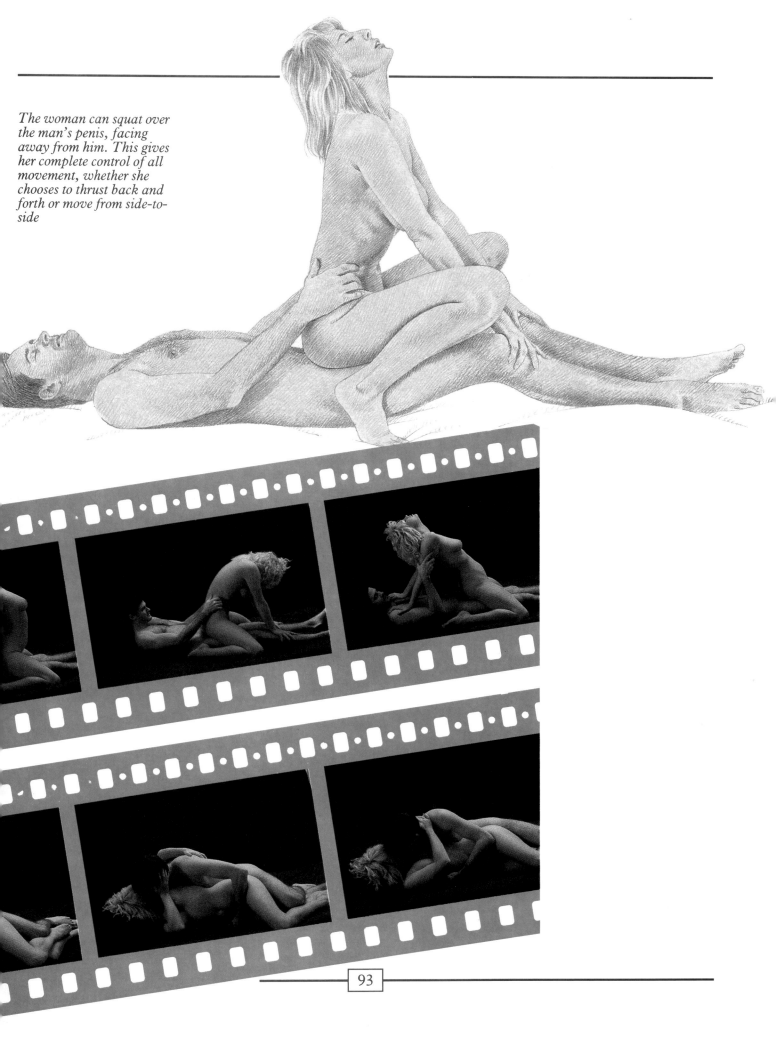

The woman can squat over the man's penis, facing away from him. This gives her complete control of all movement, whether she chooses to thrust back and forth or move from side-to-side

☐ The woman lies back in a deep armchair, raises her legs and puts her ankles on the shoulders of her partner who kneels in front of her to penetrate her.

☐ The woman lies down flat on her back with her legs apart. The man is face down with his weight mainly taken on his knees and elbows.

☐ The woman lies on her side facing away from the man who lies behind her, moulding into her body contours. (This is called 'the spoons' position). These positions enable the man, especially, to control his speed to orgasm.

Positions in which the woman can move well:

☐ The woman sits astride her man's penis, facing him as he sits on an armless chair.

☐ The man lies flat on his back and the woman sits astride him facing either towards or away from his face. She can either rest on her knees or have her feet flat on the bed in a squatting position.

☐ The man kneels on the floor and then leans back to take his weight on his hands behind him. The woman squats on his penis facing him.

These positions are good for women who like to control the movement so as to produce an orgasm for themselves during intercourse.

Positions in which neither can move much:

☐ Standing positions, particularly in which the woman hangs around the man's neck and wraps her legs around his waist.

☐ The man sits on an armless chair, legs wide apart. The woman faces away from him and sits on his penis.

☐ The man lies flat on his back with his legs together.

The woman kneels over his penis facing his feet.

☐ The woman lies on her back, legs drawn up, feet flat on the bed or held up by grasping behind the knees. The man is on his side at right angles to her body as he penetrates her. This is an exceptionally good position for teaching a woman to have an orgasm during intercourse, because it enables the man to caress her clitoris and breasts easily during penetration.

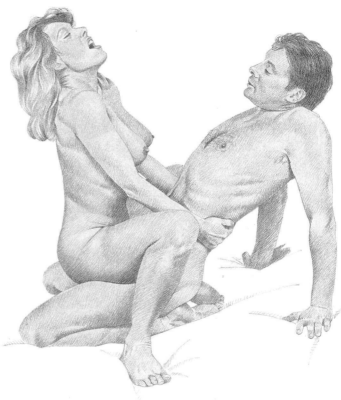

Here, the man supports himself as he kneels with the woman sitting astride him, face-to-face. Her scope for side movement, however, is somewhat limited

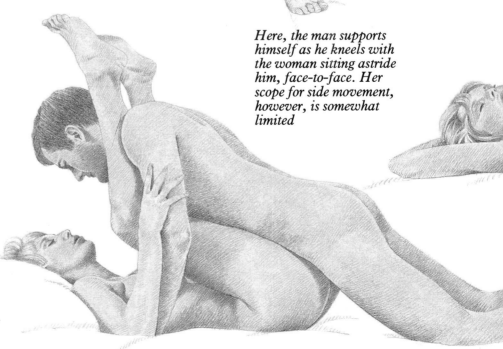

To allow the man uninhibited movement – and deep penetration – the woman bends her knees and puts both ankles over his shoulders

These positions are especially good for the couple who enjoy stimulating the man by contracting the woman's vaginal muscles rather than by a series of general body movements.

THRUSTING MOVEMENTS

As well as varying their positions for lovemaking, a couple can also vary the thrusting movements they use during sex. Couples who both like to take an active role in thrusting can try the following routines and discover which movements please each other best.

☐ Once the man has penetrated his partner, he should withdraw a little. The woman then pushes against his penis and withdraws a little. The couple should continue this alternate movement until they reach orgasm.

☐ Or, if they prefer, the couple can move simul-taneously, coming together and then withdrawing a little, but all the time with the man penetrating his partner. With both these routines, it takes a little time to perfect the rhythm.

By varying his thrusting movement, the man can greatly increase his partner's pleasure:

☐ For maximum penetration and friction, he can enter his partner, and as well as thrusting in and out, can also thrust to right and left.

☐ Another technique to maximize friction is if the man partly inserts his penis into his partner's vagina and thrusts in and out, using short strokes, before plunging his penis in up to the root.

☐ For maximum penetration, the man can enter his partner fully so that their pubic hairs are touching and then attempt a thrusting movement without withdrawing his penis at all.

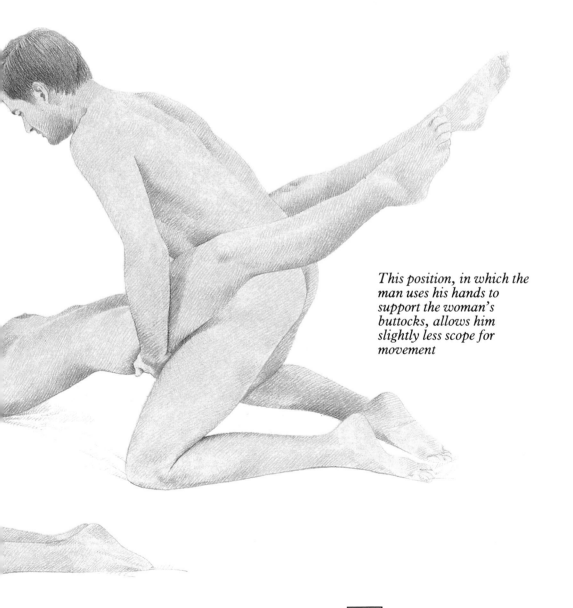

This position, in which the man uses his hands to support the woman's buttocks, allows him slightly less scope for movement

HOW TO SEDUCE YOUR WIFE

Seducing a woman is always a challenge for some men, but seducing a long-term partner can be an occasion which brings even greater rewards

---

After a few years of marriage or living together, some couples find that sex and intimacy lose their original sparkle and that they drift into a routine of day-to-day lovemaking that lacks imagination and excitement. This does not mean that their sex lives need a drastic overhaul, but it is an excellent idea to add something extra from time to time, to make lovemaking particularly enjoyable.

A NEW LOVE AFFAIR

A good way of doing this, and one which works whatever the length of your relationship, is to make a positive effort to seduce your partner and to forget that you are 'old hands' at the game of love. This has many unexpected side effects and can keep an otherwise ordinary sex life alive year after year, to the delight of you both.

Most people associate seduction with new love affairs but this need not be so. If you are planning to seduce a long-term partner, however, it makes sense to build your seduction into an organized event, especially as many women are so delighted by romance and anticipation.

PREPARE WELL AHEAD

We all enjoy special occasions, and given that anticipation is half the fun, it is sensible to plan your seduction well in advance. Indeed, some people enjoy the preparation every bit as much as the seduction itself.

By preparing well ahead, you stand the best possible chance of everything going well with your seduction.

If you have any children, arrange a babysitter in advance so that there will be no last-minute surprises.

Book up the places you intend to go. If you decide to go out for a meal, be sure to book so that you have the best chance of going exactly where your wife would most enjoy. If you are going to see a film or a show in the afternoon, then book this up too.

The real seducer leaves nothing to chance –

uncertainty and let-downs are a great turn-off. Also, your wife will be delighted to think that you have gone to all this trouble for her. By planning ahead you will be able to relax on the day and so leave yourself really free to enjoy the seduction, rather than worrying about whether everything will work out right.

PUT HER NEEDS FIRST

Buy her a little present of some kind – perhaps some favourite perfume or some sexy underwear. Also, to add spice to the night, you can visit a sex shop and buy a sex enhancer, such as a vibrator, which you can introduce as an appropriate moment during the seduction scene.

Whatever you buy, be sure that it will please her, not just yourself. She is the important person in the seduction, so put your needs second.

If you are well prepared, the day itself will be all the more pleasurable for you both.

ON THE DAY

How much of your plan you want to divulge and how much you will keep as a surprise is, of course, up to you, but most couples like at least some of the planned activities to remain secret.

A good warm-up to a seduction evening is to do something non-sexual together in the afternoon. Go to a romantic film, perhaps have a walk in the country together – all these work wonders at building up a level of intimacy between you as you unwind from the pressures of family and working life. This time is essential because few people, especially parents of small children, can switch readily from family responsibilities to uninhibited sexuality.

Unless you have a time of non-sexual intimacy together, much of your efforts at seducing your wife could be wasted and frustrating for you both.

BECOME RELAXED

Nothing you do should be too exhausting. Do not wear yourselves out doing something too vigorous if

---

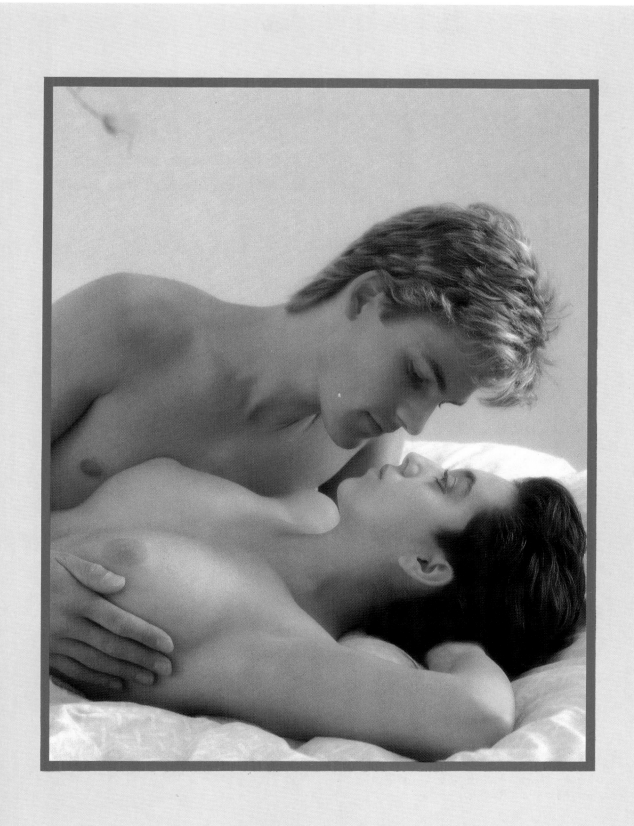

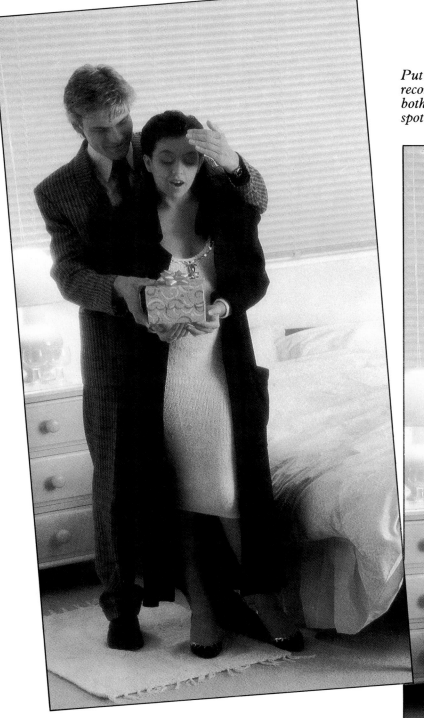

Put on a piece of your favourite music, preferably a record that will bring back romantic memories for you both. Dance closely – you hardly need move from the spot – and whisper words of love in her ear

Save your present until you have returned home after dinner – this is the time she would least expect it. Whatever you give, wrap it prettily and she will appreciate the efforts you have made

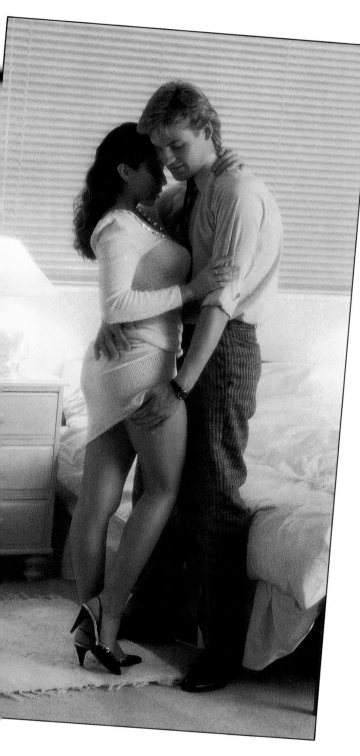

The closeness, the music and the atmosphere will almost certainly have aroused her, and now is the time to make your caress a little more sensual – but take your time as you still have a long way to go. When the moment is appropriate, you can both head for the bedroom, ready for more intimate contact.

you plan a seductive evening together, or one or both of you may fall asleep and ruin your plans.

After your quiet, intimate time together, go home and prepare for the evening. Spend some time washing, bathing or showering, so that you are clean and fresh for what is to follow. Take special care of your hair and nails, clean your teeth and ensure that your genital area is clean.

SET THE MOOD

Some couples greatly enjoy doing all this together, showering one another and so on, but others like to do things separately and present themselves 'ready for action' after a private time alone. It is simply a matter of choice and this can change from time to time in any relationship.

Ideally it is best to go out to dinner. This is a way of relaxing, gives you a chance to share things with each other and to enjoy each other as lovers, not as parents and householders. Make a real effort not to discuss the children, the mortgage or the leaking garage roof. Talk about yourselves in a caring and loving way and flirt with each other.

AN INTIMATE DINNER

If the place you go to eat can also include dancing, so much the better. Dancing is really a form of foreplay when it takes place between lovers.

During the meal, be sure not to eat or drink too much. No one feels very seductive or, indeed, likes being seduced, if they are drunk or have indigestion.

And be sensitive about what you eat. If one of you wants a dish with garlic in it, it makes sense that the other has something with garlic too, or the evening could be less than romantic right from the start. Certain foods are especially sexy to eat and a seductive man can make the most of this. Give your wife little tastes of your dishes and get her to do the same. This will create a feeling of intimacy between you.

Use the meal to talk sweet nothings to her. Chat her up as you would a new partner.

Compliment her on her hair, her eyes, her looks generally and praise whatever features you can with honesty. Try being really uninhibited about saying loving things to her. Make her feel really wanted and loved and tell her how much she means to you.

On your return home, continue to be exceptionally attentive and loving towards her; once there you might continue the mood by putting on a favourite piece of music to set a more romantic and conducive mood.

THE SEDUCTION

So far, apart from the dancing, there has probably been little very intimate physical contact. However, your partner may already feel highly sexy and be very amorous indeed. The compliments, the time together, the effort you have put into it all, and the pure

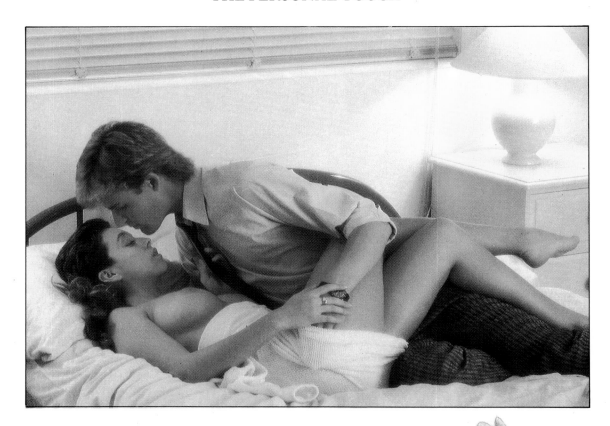

(above) Don't rush things, gradually remove both of your clothes bit by bit, pausing to fondle your wife's body. Take time to tell her how much the sight of her arouses you

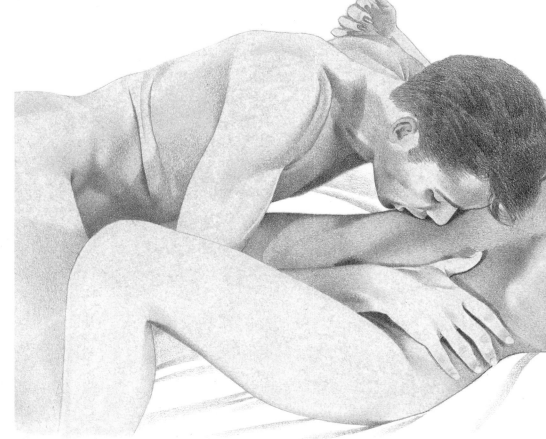

(right) Remember, you can use your mouth as well as your hands to caress and tease the whole of her body

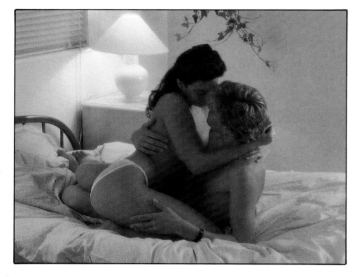

relaxation of doing nice things will probably have aroused her and taken her back to your courtship days and previous romantic interludes.

Only now does the sexual side of the seduction begin, but the job is already more than half done.

DANCE TOGETHER
Start by dancing together. Turn the lights down low, put on some favourite music and just spend time dancing closely and being in one another's arms. Kiss a lot and snuggle into one another. Take it gently and do not go straight for intercourse. She may ask you to make love to her – but do not do so.

REMOVE HER CLOTHES
Instead, slowly undress her as you dance and compliment her on her beautiful body. Tell her how much it turns you on.

Take as much time as you like for kisses, caresses and words of love. This type of non-genital contact will greatly heighten the pleasures you feel when you eventually make love and almost certainly improve the quality of your orgasm

Keep close together – skin-to-skin contact enhances the feeling of emotional closeness. Holding hands in this situation can say more than the most eloquent declaration of love

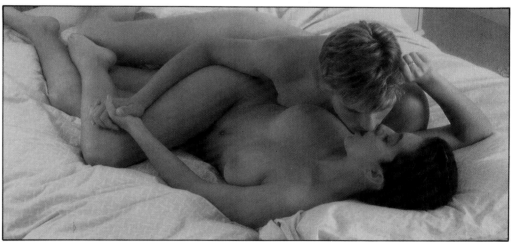

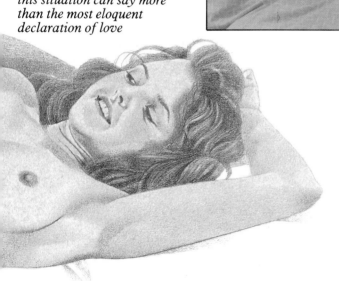

At this point, you will probably both want to retire to your bedroom, so make sure that you have prepared the room and the things you will need before you go out. And remember to leave the heating on so that the room is warm and cosy.

If she is still partly clothed, put on some music and ask her to strip for you. This should be a real turn-on for her as well as you unless she is exceptionally inhibited, because many women are exhibitionists at heart and enjoy showing off to their lovers.

COURTSHIP GAMES
Once she is stripped, you can give her the sexy undies and ask her to try them on. Get her to model them as if she were in a fashion show. At this stage, resurrect any sexual games you played in your courtship days. Many couples remember them with affection and the silliness of the situation heightens their pleasure in each other.

FOREPLAY
If the seduction is going well, now is the time to take things a stage further. A woman who is aroused by all

this sensuality and preparation will almost certainly feel less inhibited than normal and will therefore be more likely to experiment sexually and be receptive to some sensually erotic massage.

Ask her to lie back with her legs apart and slowly caress her body from top to toe. Massage her, if she likes this, preferably using some scented massage oil. Tease her breasts and nipples and intimately massage all the parts of her body that you know excite her.

Now caress her vulva and clitoris so that she is

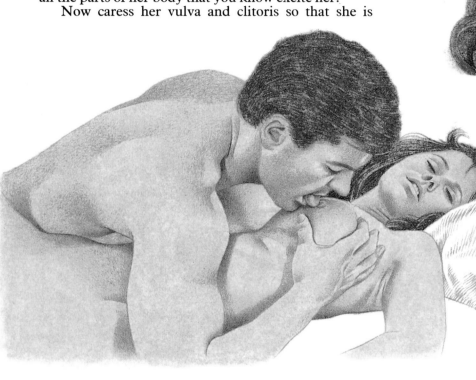

If your partner has sensitive breasts, spend some time leisurely licking, sucking and kissing her nipples – you will probably find this activity every bit as pleasurable as she will

highly aroused. All the time encourage her to do to you whatever you know she enjoys best. Remember that you are seducing her and enabling her to get the best out of it. It is not an excuse for you to be selfish at her expense.

When she is highly aroused and well lubricated, insert first one finger and then two and do whatever she likes best with them. Some women like them to be thrust in and out like a penis, others like their G spot stimulated, others their cervix played with and moved about, and yet others enjoy having the fingers kept still. If you don't know, ask her.

USE THE VIBRATOR

As the tension mounts you can bring out the vibrator. Have it ready somewhere handy so that you do not have to break off the flow of loving talk and caresses. Slowly insert it in to her vagina a little at a time. She may be amazed at the new sensation and will want to know what is going on. If you think from your previous knowledge of her she will enjoy it, show it to her and tell what you are going to do with it.

Use the vibrator exactly as she wants and be guided by her body movements and unspoken messages as to

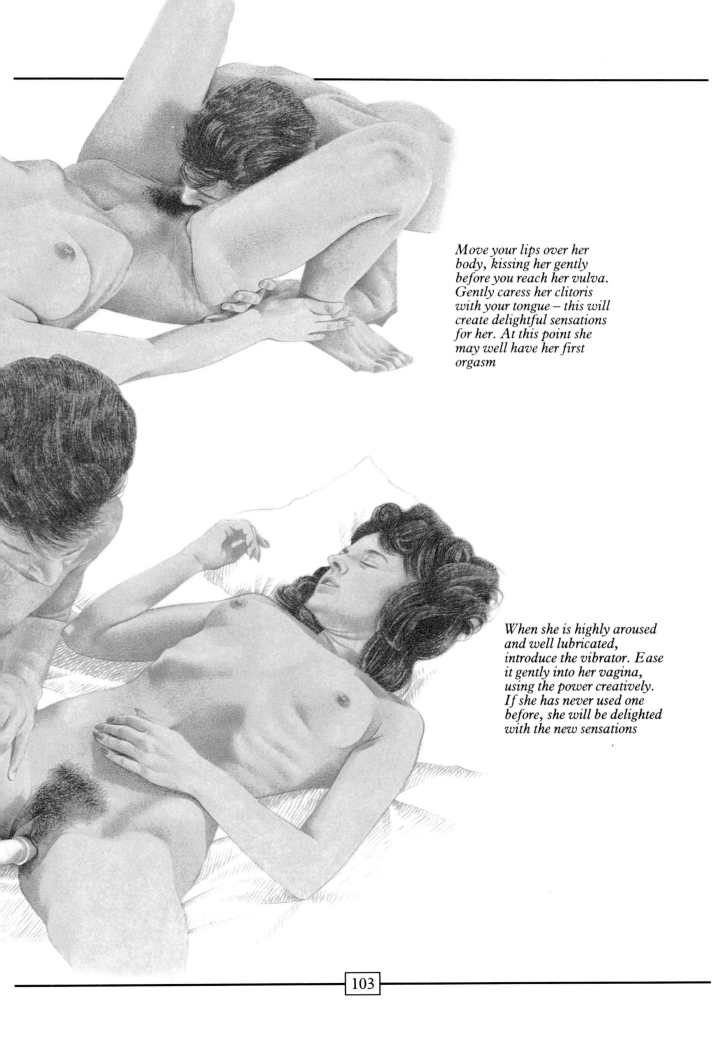

Move your lips over her body, kissing her gently before you reach her vulva. Gently caress her clitoris with your tongue – this will create delightful sensations for her. At this point she may well have her first orgasm

When she is highly aroused and well lubricated, introduce the vibrator. Ease it gently into her vagina, using the power creatively. If she has never used one before, she will be delighted with the new sensations

what she best likes. She may not know what is best if it is a new experience, so you will have to play it by ear and offer her initial variety.

MAKE LOVE

By now, she will be highly excited and will probably want you to make love to her. Now is a good time to try a new or unorthodox position that produces a new sensation for her.

Alternatively, she could have her first orgasm with the vibrator inside her vagina while you pay special attention to other parts of her body.

Even if she usually has only one orgasm, she will, after all this build-up, be more than ready to make love in one of her favourite positions. If she is normally multi-orgasmic, however, she will experience more orgasms as you have intercourse with her, or alternatively a particularly enjoyable one if she usually has just the one.

AND AFTERWARDS

When you have finished making love, let your wife decide what a perfect end to the evening would be. She may well want to fall asleep in your arms or she might want to talk about something that is loving and intimate for you both. If you do have a chance to talk before you fall asleep, tell her how much you need her. Most women love to hear that they are wanted and

desired, not just that they are loved by their husbands.

Tell her what you most enjoyed and why, especially if it was something new and perhaps daring for her. Encourage her to talk about her best pleasures of the time you had together – they may have been something you did in the afternoon together, or a part of the meal out, perhaps the dancing. Remember what she says so that you can build the experience into your next act of seduction.

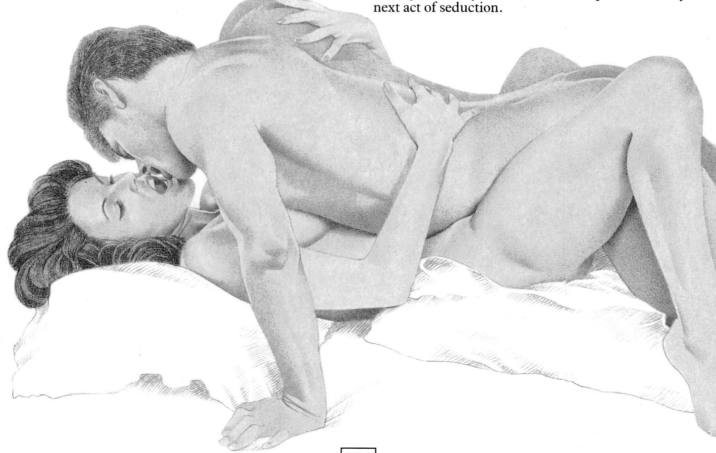

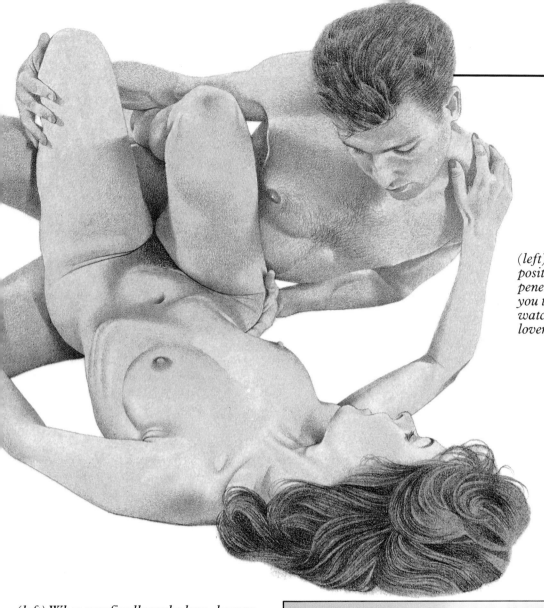

(left) Adopting a side position like this, to penetrate your wife, allows you to see her face and watch her response to your lovemaking

(below) Once you have both enjoyed your orgasm, lie close together and take time to talk – this is an occasion when afterplay is all-important and it may well be that it will set the scene for another bout of lovemaking

(left) When you finally make love, be sure it is an unhurried and relaxed affair – avoid deep and urgent thrusting movements and keep the pace slow until you both feel you are ready for orgasm. You can then speed up the action

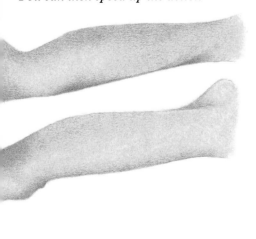

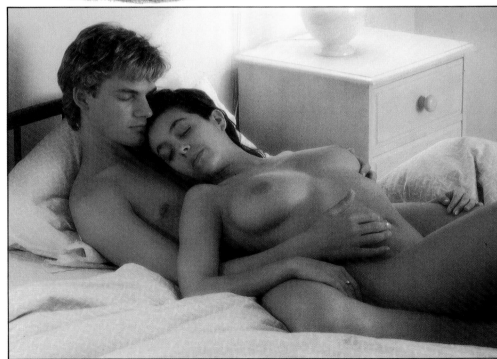

HOW TO SEDUCE YOUR HUSBAND

Seducing your husband may seem a novel idea, but it can pay dividends in terms of your relationship and add something special to your sex life

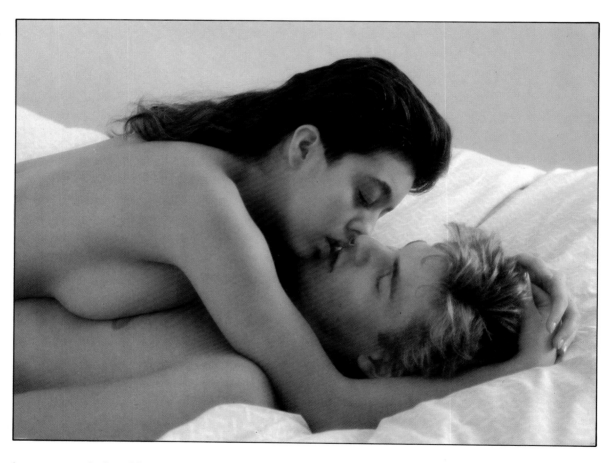

I n any long-term relationship, the man as well as the woman can feel that he is taken for granted from time to time. And even if the sexual side of the relationship is satisfactory, the act of intercourse can all too easily become more of a duty than a pleasure.

Setting out actively to seduce your husband is a worthwhile exercise, especially as most men are more easily seduced than women. The promise of sex with someone they love is often enough to excite them, but the build-up to a seduction can increase the pleasure.

Let your husband know that you mean to use your whole body to give him his most memorable sexual experience ever

THE BENEFITS OF FAMILIARITY

In the early days of a relationship, finding 'new' ways to please a partner in bed is scarcely necessary. At that time, sex is always exciting, always different. The reasons for this are partly that the couple are unfamiliar with each other, and much of their pleasure is derived from the novelty of sex with a new partner.

Also, when a couple first find love, they can barely wait to see each other, not just to make love, but to kiss, touch and talk. For a period of time, life is full of sensations of surprise and anticipation.

When the couple have been together for some time, the initial feelings of excitement dull, sex is no longer new and familiarity sets in. But familiarity can be a powerful weapon and can be used to good effect in an act of seduction. The woman who knows her partner's body and knows what he likes having done to him, can give him maximum pleasure without going through the process of trial and error.

TACTICS NOT STRATEGY

The tactics a woman employs to seduce her husband are all-important. Although there is only one purpose, to please and pamper your man in a way that is exclusively pleasurable to him, the route taken to that point is variable. For most men, sex is something that is better when it is dressed up. The dressing can be words, a mood, clothes, a new place to make love, almost anything that you want. The aim is to give your husband a perfect evening.

SETTING THE MOOD

Sex or sexual intercourse is only part of the seduction, and as with any event, a large part of the excitement is in the preparation.

PREPARATION

It is a good idea to make a list, planning what you intend to do. Cooking one of his favourite meals is probably a better option than taking him out to dinner. The preparation need not be fiddly, and a cold supper will mean that the time you eat is not too crucial. This could be important if your plans go astray and the meal is delayed.

Decide whether you are going to let him know what you intend to do, or whether you want it to be a surprise. A good compromise is to ring him up at work on the day and tell him that you have something very special ready for him that evening.

As the emphasis of the evening is to be on sex, hiring a sexy video may be a good idea. You can hire one, especially a favourite one, from your local video shop the day before the event.

Take time to decide what you are going to wear. The way you dress, and therefore the way you look, are the most visible means of arousing a man and the right attire can make all the difference between a succesful seduction and an ordinary evening.

CHOOSE WITH CARE

This is his special evening so choose whatever you know will turn him on. Try to be sensitive to his needs. Some men may like black underwear, stockings and suspenders with high-heeled shoes, others may

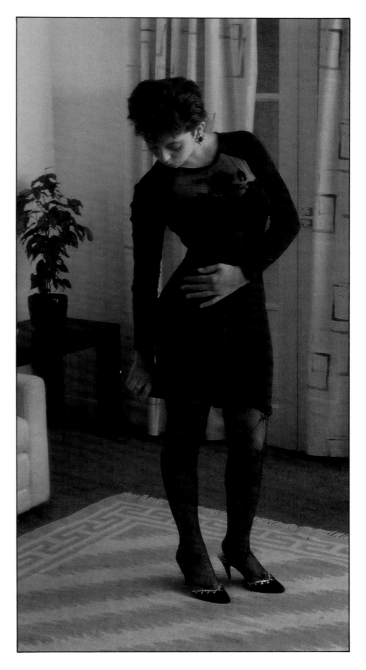

On the evening, choose something to wear which you know your husband will find particularly sexy. Take your time and watch yourself as you dress

prefer pure white, virginal underwear – and the demure-looking virgin who turns into a whore is many a man's sexual fantasy.

Make sure that whatever you choose is easy to remove. Many an ardent lover has lost his control, or even his erection, while undoing rows of tiny buttons.

Finally, give some thought to exactly how you are going to carry out the seduction and exactly what you intend to do to your husband to make this the most memorable seduction he has ever experienced.

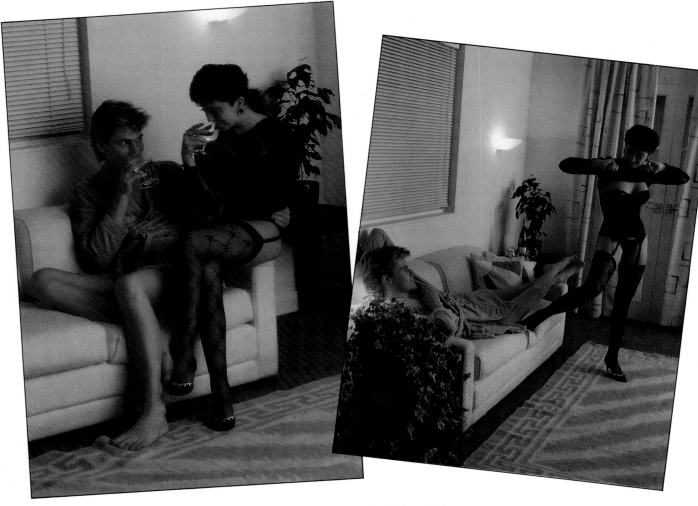

ON THE DAY

Creating an atmosphere for seduction is of prime importance on the day. If you intend to extend your lovemaking throughout the house, make sure the heating is turned up – a chilly house can cool the ardour of even the most aroused lover.

If you intend to have wine, or better still champagne, make sure it is chilled and ready to serve at the right temperature.

Finally, get yourself in the mood for love. Once the meal is prepared, languish in a hot, scented bath and think about the evening ahead with anticipation. The mere thought of what is going to happen should begin to make you feel highly sexy.

Before you dress, let yourself relax for a time, wrapped only in a towel. Perhaps having a sneak preview of the evening's entertainment will also increase your sexual awareness. Put the video on and watch a little bit. If you feel like it, lie on the sofa and masturbate – a taste of orgasm will almost certainly put you in the mood for more.

Take your time to dress. If you have a full-length mirror, watch yourself as you start to cover your body – if you look good you will almost certainly feel good

(left) Partially strip and then relax with a drink. Sit close to your husband – with your arms around him

(above) Put some music on and start removing the rest of your clothes. Tease your husband by letting him caress you from time to time, but let it go no further than a touch

(right) Once you have removed all your clothes, you can help your husband out of his robe. By this time you should both be feeling aroused and ready for action

about yourself and be in just the right mood when your husband arrives home.

THE SEDUCTION

After a hard day at work, an early-evening bath is one of the most sensuous ways of relaxing. Run a hot bath for your husband, filling it with fragrant bath oil.

When he arrives home, greet him at the door, take him inside and pour him his favourite drink. Then escort him into the bathroom, undress him, help him into the bath and leave his drink within easy reach.

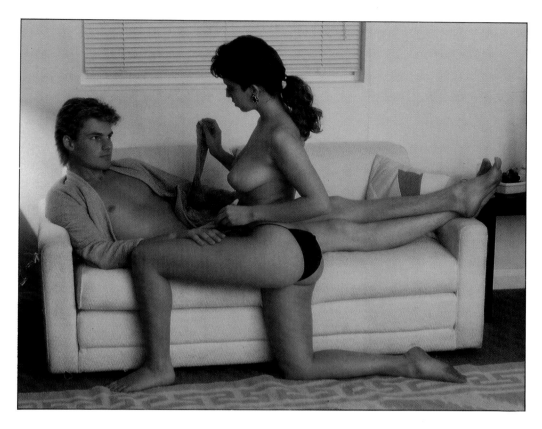

Take your dress off so you do not get it wet. This will let him see what you are wearing underneath. If you feel like it, remove your panties and 'forget' to put them on again before dinner. This should give him more than a hint of what is in store later.

A TASTE OF THINGS TO COME
You will know your husband's sexual capabilities and how many times he is capable of reaching orgasm in any love-making session. Most men, however, provided the stimulus is high, are capable of having at least two orgasms during an evening.

With your husband still in the bath, tell him to close his eyes and take his penis in your hands. Gently rub each testicle and run your hands up and down the penis shaft. To add to the sensuality, use both hands slowly at first, building up to an insistent rhythm.

Tell him how desirable you find him and whether you are going to make him come. Praise his body and tell him how powerful his orgasm will be. There is nothing that he needs to do except to lie back and enjoy what is happening to him.

Build up the speed at which your hands move until he achieves orgasm.

When he has recovered, dry him off and help him into a bathrobe – there will be no need for him to dress again on this particular evening.

THE MEAL
During the meal, give him your full attention and use the time to spoil him thoroughly. Keep his wine glass full but do not overdo the drinks for either him or yourself. Because the imagination is so strong, tell him some of what you intend to do later.

Once you have finished the meal, take him by the hand to the living room and switch on the erotic video.

WATCHING THE VIDEO
Nestle up to him or lie in his lap as you both watch the video. When you find any scene particularly stimulating or exciting, place your hand under his robe and, almost absentmindedly, rub his penis. If you are feeling aroused yourself, place his hand under your dress so that he can feel your clitoris. At this stage, resist any insistence he may make to make love. There will be plenty of time later.

AROUSAL
When the video is over, or when you feel that you are both sufficiently aroused, switch the video off and stand up. Tell your husband to relax, put on a favourite piece of music, dim the lights and take your clothes off in front of him. If you have decided to wear stockings and suspenders, keep those on. Do not hurry removing your clothes and move to the music. When they are all off, touch yourself and stimulate your clitoris. Move up to him and use your breasts to tease and tantalize him. Let him touch you but never for too long, always moving away if he becomes too insistent. The idea is to stir him, making him fully aware of every part of your body, and thus raising the sexual temperature.

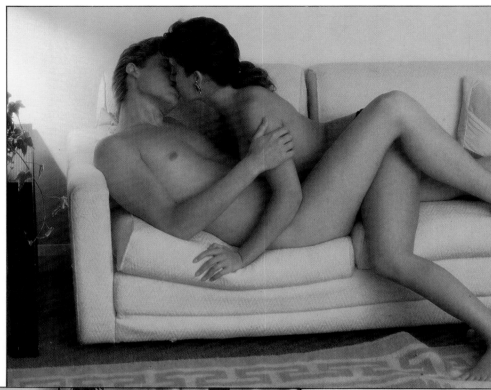

When you are both naked, take time to kiss. Use your tongue imaginatively and do not restrict your kisses to his mouth

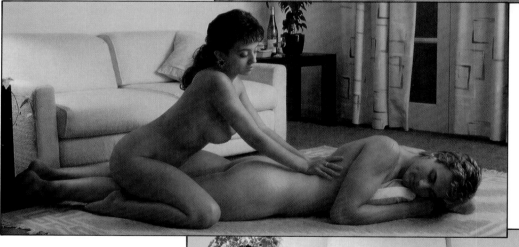

Now is the time to treat your man to an erotic massage. Ask him exactly which areas he would most like you to pay attention to

When you finally get down to intercourse, take the initiative and make love to him in a woman-on-top position. This will really show that you are intent on pleasuring him

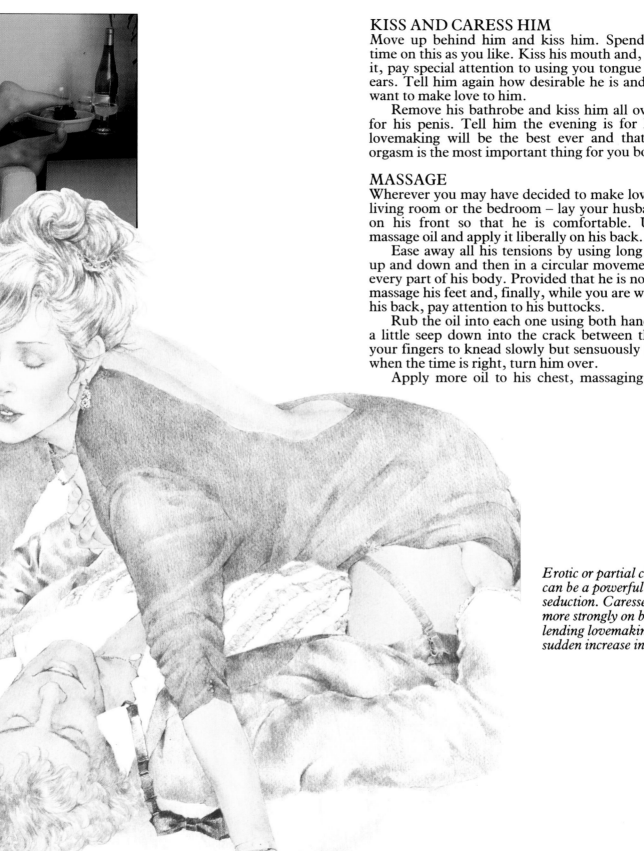

KISS AND CARESS HIM

Move up behind him and kiss him. Spend as much time on this as you like. Kiss his mouth and, if he likes it, pay special attention to using you tongue inside his ears. Tell him again how desirable he is and how you want to make love to him.

Remove his bathrobe and kiss him all over except for his penis. Tell him the evening is for him, that lovemaking will be the best ever and that his own orgasm is the most important thing for you both.

MASSAGE

Wherever you may have decided to make love – in the living room or the bedroom – lay your husband down on his front so that he is comfortable. Use some massage oil and apply it liberally on his back.

Ease away all his tensions by using long strokes – up and down and then in a circular movement. Cover every part of his body. Provided that he is not ticklish, massage his feet and, finally, while you are working on his back, pay attention to his buttocks.

Rub the oil into each one using both hands and let a little seep down into the crack between them. Use your fingers to knead slowly but sensuously and then, when the time is right, turn him over.

Apply more oil to his chest, massaging it slowly

Erotic or partial clothing can be a powerful tool in a seduction. Caresses are felt more strongly on bare flesh, lending lovemaking a sudden increase in urgency

but firmly. As well as your hands, use your breasts to apply the oil. Most men are more genitally sensitive than women so do not leave it too long before your pay his penis some attention. Massage his legs and thighs, but do not put any oil on his penis yet.

WORSHIP THE PENIS

For the woman who is happy giving oral sex to her husband, now is the time to use your mouth as sensually as you know how on his penis. This is an act of lovemaking which few men can resist.

Make yourself as comfortable as you can and use your tongue on his testicles and then slowly lick along the length of his penis. Use one of your hands to encircle its root and take it into mouth as far as you can. Move your head up and down and use the other hand to stroke his body elsewhere as you suck.

Here again your own body will serve to increase his arousal still further. As you move your mouth on his penis, shift your bottom so that it is over his face. Use your vulva to give him a full genital kiss, moving it from side to side as he uses his tongue on you. Use the pressure of your body to hold him down.

This will serve to arouse him still further and as the tempo increases, concentrate on making it the most memorable experience of oral sex that he has ever had.

Refuse all pleas to let him come inside your mouth unless that is what you have both decided upon, and when you sense that the time is right, lift your vulva away from his mouth and turn round.

MAKE LOVE

The woman-on-top position where you face your husband, is probably the position you should choose to finish off his seduction.

This enables him to see exactly what you are doing as you move your lower body to bring him to orgasm. Also you are free to kiss and caress him as you make love and you can also use your breasts to press against his face or he can suck your nipples as you both move towards orgasm.

Squat over his penis, rubbing it slowly against your clitoris. Move your hips around and around as you do this, then take the root of his penis in one hand and descend quickly on to it so that the penetration is as deep as you want.

Move slowly at first, up and down so that on each outward movement his penis is almost out of you, but not quite. Then sink back on to him, always trying for deeper and deeper penetration with stronger and stronger movements. To increase it still further, you can always lean forward towards him.

Now you can vary the up and down movements and move from side to side, keeping his penis deep inside you. Rub your clitoris as you do this – your own orgasm will be important to both of you now. Vary the movements, only being consistent in quickening the speed and urgency.

Try to time your orgasm so that is coincides with his. Let him stay inside you as long as he likes.

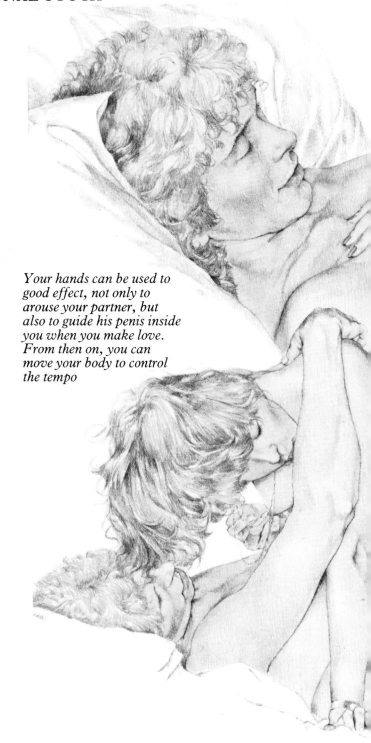

Your hands can be used to good effect, not only to arouse your partner, but also to guide his penis inside you when you make love. From then on, you can move your body to control the tempo

AND AFTERWARDS . . .

Lie with your head on his chest and tell him how marvellous it was for you. Use your tongue on his chest and stomach and snuggle up to him. If he wants to sleep, let him, but if you feel that he may become aroused again, remember that your own body, and your mouth particularly, may be the best means of rearousing him.

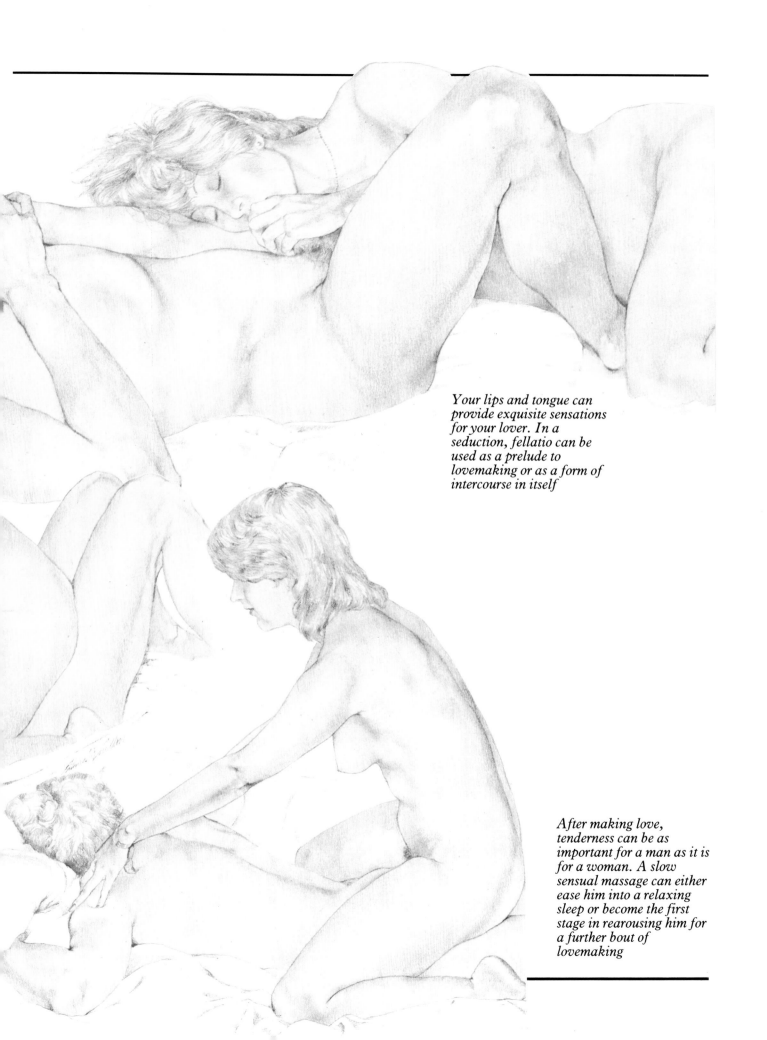

Your lips and tongue can provide exquisite sensations for your lover. In a seduction, fellatio can be used as a prelude to lovemaking or as a form of intercourse in itself

After making love, tenderness can be as important for a man as it is for a woman. A slow sensual massage can either ease him into a relaxing sleep or become the first stage in rearousing him for a further bout of lovemaking

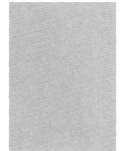
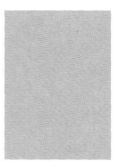

MORE ROMANTIC LOVEMAKING

With a little thought and imagination, any couple can rediscover the early romance that existed in the first weeks of their courtship. And the familiar feelings between them can be used to good effect to turn their lovemaking into memorable experience

Most of us understand romance to imply attentiveness, consideration and sensuality in a lover. It conjures up images of being in love when a relationship is new, fresh and exciting. The feelings it creates can be exquisitely insane or they may be agonizing and depressing.

THE ROMANTIC MALE
Another definition of romance is as an exaggeration or picturesque falsehood. The romantic lover includes a combination of both descriptions in his romantic behaviour, acting in a loving and attentive way but in an exaggerated manner,

Most of us start our relationships by being loving and romantic towards our partners. For the man, this may mean giving flowers or presents when they are least expected, or providing surprise meals or outings. This is standard courtship procedure.

He is attentive and communicates his feelings to his partner. He may exaggerate them, he may dress them up. Possibly he will telephone at odd moments just to say how he feels. He will make every effort to look good, and on arranged outings he will make every effort to be punctual.

A NATURAL STATE
A man may behave like this for a variety of reasons. He may want to get the woman into bed as quickly as possibly, seeing flattery as the quickest means of achieving that end. He may see himself as a James Bond character who treats women in this way. Some men see sex in terms of conquest.

But research has shown that most men actually behave romantically because they want to – they simply feel romantic and the resultant behaviour is natural and spontaneous. In a culture where literature, films and TV predominantly cater for the woman as the more romantic consumer, many men are actually surprised that women are considered to be the more romantic sex.

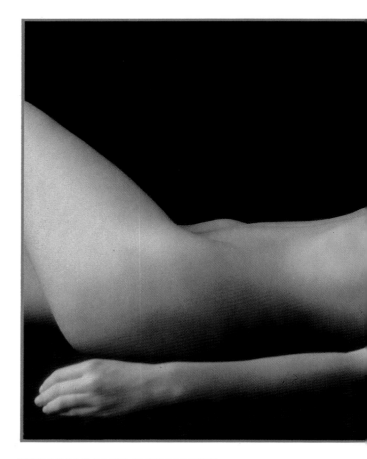

WOMAN AND ROMANCE
For most women in the very early days of a relationship, romance is something that they feel rather than a way they behave. This is partly because our culture still expects men to make the first move.

But romance is an addictive drug and does not depend only on actions. More important and potent are the feelings it creates.

In the early stages of a relationship, it is these

romantic feelings that dictate the way a woman behaves in much the same way they do for a man. And whether it is through the way she dresses, the gifts she presents or the passion of the early physical contact, she sees her partner through rose-tinted glasses in the same way that he sees her.

And just as he credits her with almost unreal qualities of sensuality and beauty, she may see in him the qualities of some fantasy lover who has before only existed in her mind.

HOW THE RECIPIENT FEELS
The reasons why we behave like this are probably less important than the actual behaviour and its effects on both ourselves and our partners.

Everyone is susceptible to flattery, presents and

Taking time in lovemaking to talk about your feelings for one another will enhance the romance of the occasion

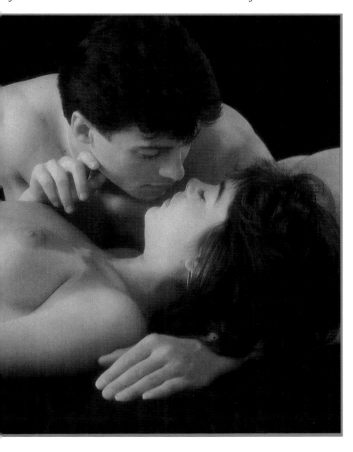

attentive behaviour. They make us feel good, prized and loved. If everything turns sour later on, the pain can be intense and long lasting, but the memories of romantic love are among the most powerful we have and remain with us for the rest of our lives.

WHEN ROMANCE GOES
Unfortunately, romantic behaviour disappears all too quickly in most long-term relationships.

Yet, this is not necessarily a bad thing. Most relationships are unable to withstand the dreamy, almost unreal quality on a permanent basis. And as a relationship progresses, the romantic qualities are replaced by something more worthwhile and much deeper, based on trust.

THE IMPORTANCE OF ROMANCE
Most people who are in a long-term relationship remember wistfully the first days of their courtship. And why not? That was the time they yearned to be together all the time. Absences were agonizing and the sex – whatever it may have lacked in finesse – was as frequent as the couple could manage.

Even when they were not making love, they were touching, kissing and cuddling. Young lovers are unable, often to the consternation of their elders, to keep their hands off each other.

Those early feelings we have for our partners are indispensable. For most people, they are the basis on which they choose to form their relationships. The love they feel may be the vital ingredient, but that in itself is often a direct result of this early romantic behaviour, which is spontaneous emotion.

FROM TIME TO TIME
In an ideal world the climate would continue to be one where romantic lovemaking goes on all the time. For most of us, however, the practicalities of life mean that we cannot continue in that vein, but the effort made to restore some romance into our relationship will be amply rewarded.

For the woman, it means being treated as someone special again, someone who is cosseted and prized. For the man, it revives his ideas of his masculinity, making him feel someone who is both loved and desired.

For both, a return to romance means not only a return to more loving behaviour, but more frequent, satisfactory sex.

ACT ROMANTICALLY

In a long-term relationship, keeping romance alive can present difficulties after the first flush of enthusiasm has waned.

Yet the couple who are in tune with one another should be able to readily recall the emotions and actions they used when they first started courting each other. The familiarity that now exists can be used to good effect. All that is needed . is thought and imagination.

☐ **Practice the art of surprise** This need not be confined to gifts such as flowers or the occasional present. A meal at a restaurant, or just a specially-cooked meal at home, can provide the right atmosphere for love. Candles, a favourite piece of music and a bottle of wine are the icing on the cake for any pair of lovers, and set the ambience and tone for the evening – and are all better if the partner on the receiving end is surprised.

☐ **Dress up from time to time** For a man, to see his partner dressed sexily is not just a turn-on, it is extremely flattering as well. It does not have to be overtly sexy, but most men are susceptible to the idea that a woman has dressed specifically for him. Equally for a man, making an effort to look good is a compliment to the woman he is with.

☐ **Act like lovers** Telephone each other from time to time just to say 'I love you'. Don't be afraid to show affection to each other in public. Even something as simple as taking your partner's hand can turn a walk into a romantic episode.

☐ **Try to recapture the mood of your courtship.** This means finding more time to spend together. A short holiday away, even a day out or perhaps revising

places that were particularly memorable to you both, can be a real tonic.

☐ **Always remember birthdays and anniversaries** It is not so much the present, but the fact that you show that you remember that counts. If possible, celebrate them with a meal or an outing.

☐ **Be more considerate** Try acting more selflessly – placing a towel on the radiator before your partner has a bath, or bringing an unexpected cup of tea in the morning, are both ways of saying 'I love you'.

☐ **Share activities more** Daily, domestic chores or shared hobbies and sports can be romantic in the right setting. Even painting and decorating, or other household improvements, can be a shared experience between lovers if the mood of both partners is right.

☐ **Touch more** A brief caress, holding hands or a touch on the shoulder does not need to have any sexual

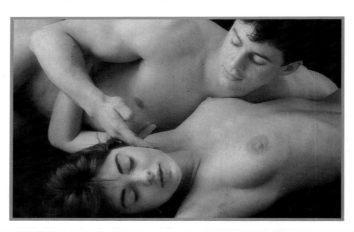

(right) Slowly caress your partner's face and neck. Spend time thinking about how much she means to you

(below) Gently move your hands over her body. Tenderly stroke and squeeze her breasts while you lightly brush your lips over her skin

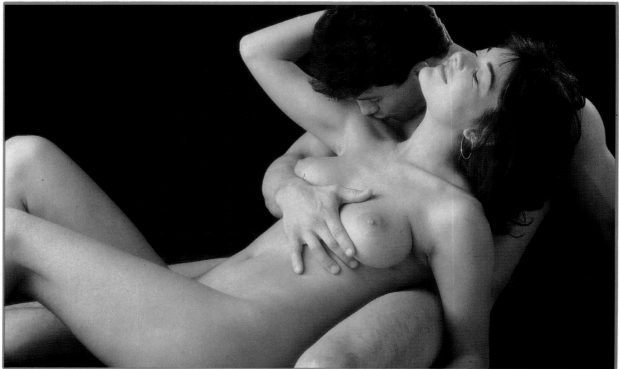

meaning and are often capable of saying 'I love you' more fluently than mere words.

☐ **Kiss and cuddle more** Do not be afraid to show each other affection – wherever you may be. Many men often think sex should really result from kissing and cuddlings. Yet often they can be an end in themselves.

☐ **Find new places to make love** Almost any room can be romantic for making love if the mood is right. But do not confine yourselves to indoors. The garden, provided it is closed to prying eyes, can be a wonderful venue on a warm evening. For the adventurous, a journey back to a place where the lovemaking has been truly memorable can provide the perfect setting.

They know exactly what turns the other on.

Although it is all too easy to fall into the routine of doing only what you know your partner likes, sex and lovemaking can be much more fun – and more romantic – if both partners explore each other's likes and dislikes, lingering over them, rather than hurrying through them.

PREPARING TO LOVE

A long, warm bath together always acts as a wonderful prelude to lovemaking. And a romantic alternative to bathing together is for each partner to bathe the other, soaping them down gently, but leaving the most sensitive of their erogenous zones until last.

MAKING LOVE ALL DAY

When it comes to romantic sex, a couple who have been together for any length of time have a collossal advantage over a couple who are just starting out together. They know each other's likes or dislikes.

ROMANTIC LOVING – HIM TO HER

For the man who really wants to go to town, take lighted candles into the bathroom to provide sensual lighting – flickering and romantic. Prepare the room you intend to make love in beforehand, perhaps

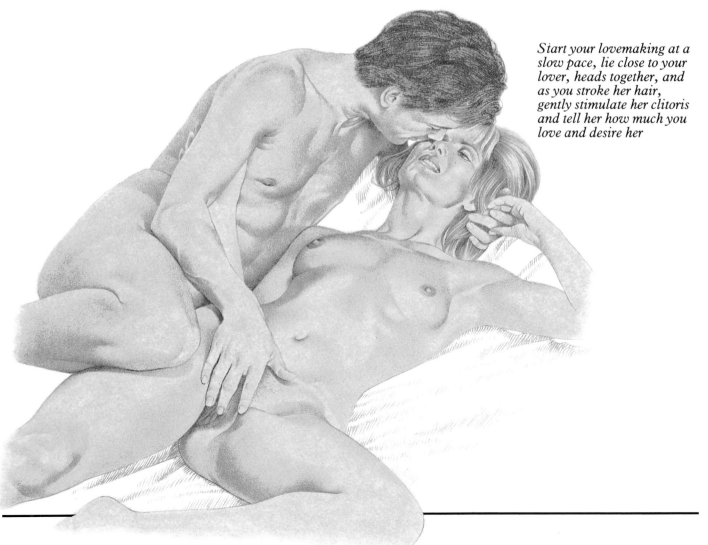

Start your lovemaking at a slow pace, lie close to your lover, heads together, and as you stroke her hair, gently stimulate her clitoris and tell her how much you love and desire her

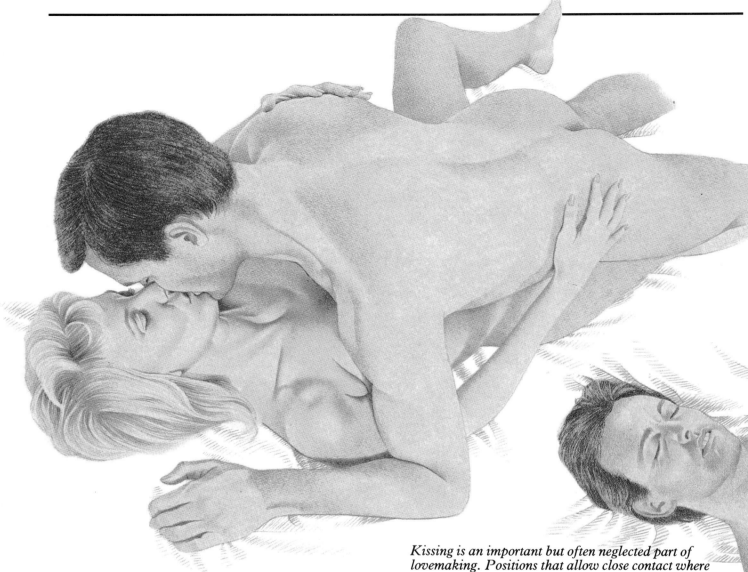

Kissing is an important but often neglected part of lovemaking. Positions that allow close contact where a couple can observe and communicate with each other help create a feeling of intimacy

leaving two glasses of your favourite wine by the bed.

Add fragrant oils to the bath as you run the water. Then take your partner into the bathroom and slowly undress her.

A SENSUAL BATH
Start by washing her shoulders, kneading them gently and using the soap as a massage oil. Move your hands down her back, using long slow strokes. Tell her how much you love her, complimenting her all the time and lingering over each hand movement. Do not be tempted to hurry – on this occasion you have all the time in the world to build an atmosphere.

Next, lie her back in the water and wash each arm, finishing by washing her hand, teasing each finger as you go. Lather the soap sensuously over her stomach, perhaps brushing each breast, but no more at this stage. Now, raise each leg out of the water separately and soap it down, thoroughly massaging the inner thighs and gently caressing her vulva – but only for a second.

If the size of the bath permits, ask her to turn over

and raise her buttocks above the water line and apply generous quantities of soap to her bottom. Then, slowly run a finger between her buttocks.

If she enjoys this, ask her to raise her bottom still higher and continue washing and rinsing.

Now, turn her over once more and lovingly wash each breast, teasing each nipple as you do so. After washing each area, make rinsing just as much of a sensual game as the soaping down.

When you are finished, dry her down thoroughly with a warmed towel, paying loving attention to all of her body from her hands and toes to her breasts and bottom. Continue to compliment her, and tell her what you intend to do later.

MAKE LOVE
When she is dry, pick her up and carry her to the bedroom or wherever you have chosen to make love. If you have provided a bottle of wine, pause while you both take a sip – but not for too long.

Kissing, cuddling and prolonged foreplay were habits learned early in courtship, so kiss her all over her body. Then, with her skin tingling from the effects of the bath, apply massage oil over her body. Massage her feet, her arms and hands, her back, legs and buttocks. Pay special attention to her breasts, applying generous amounts of oil to them. Massage first one breast then the other, teasing each nipple in turn.

EXPLORE HER BODY

Oral sex is often considered the greatest compliment a lover can pay to his partner.

When the oil has been massaged all over her, lay her back and find a position that is also comfortable to you. Use your tongue on her clitoris with slow, attentive strokes, moving rhythmically the way you both know that she likes it.

Tease her by darting your tongue in and out of her vagina. Tell her how you love her 'down there', and use your hands to explore the rest of her body. Bring her to the brink of orgasm.

POSITIONS

Any position that allows a couple to gaze at each other and kiss and touch can be romantic. For the man who is spoiling his partner, any of the man-on-top positions are suitable. They allow the man to feel he is in control and he can see and gauge his partner's reactions as they make love.

With your partner lying back on the bed, part her legs gently and enter her. Start off with short, shallow strokes and move slowly at first.

For the woman who wants to give her partner maximum pleasure, the first step is to watch how he masturbates, taking note of how he holds his penis, speed of his hand movement and rhythm. From there, she will be able to use her knowledge to satisfy him further.

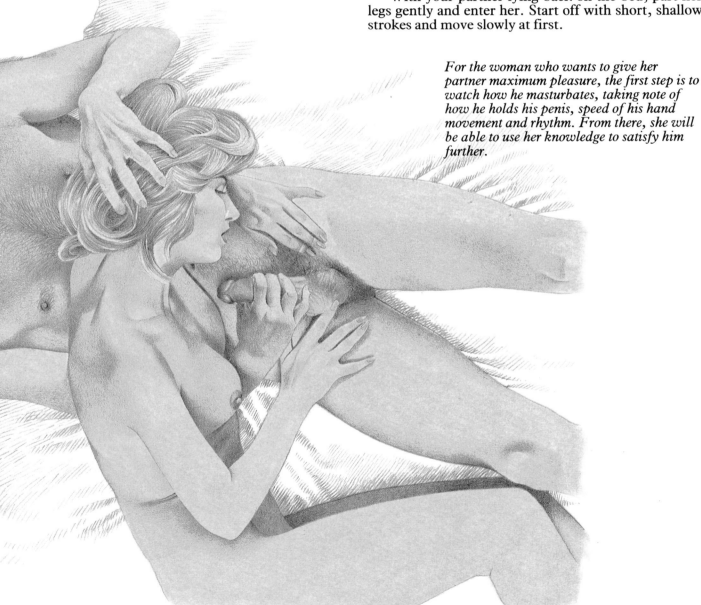

Tell her what you want to do and how you want to bring her to orgasm.

AFTERPLAY

More neglected than any other part of lovemaking, the time after orgasm can be the most implicitly romantic.

Many couples are contented to fall asleep, but as the woman relaxes in the afterglow of satisfactory sex, the man who kisses and cuddles his partner can relax and spoil her still further.

Use this as a time of physical well-being to caress your partner and then, if the mood takes you, you can always make love again.

ROMANTIC LOVING – HER TO HIM

Most men love to be bathed. Because your body will be such a turn-on for him, wear as little as possible – a pair of panties should be enough. Then undress him, pampering him like a baby. When he is lying in the bath, dangle your breasts over him for a moment, but do not let him touch them.

A UNIQUE EXPERIENCE

Start by soaping down his chest with round, sweeping strokes making as much lather as possible. Wash his arms as lovingly as he washed yours and then soap down his legs. Pay special attention to the tops of his thighs but, do not touch his penis.

Ask him to turn over and raise his bottom in the air and soap it down generously. Use a finger to wash and tease him between his buttocks, rinsing him thoroughly.

Turn him over again to wash his penis. Make a lather in his pubic hair, and gently wash his testicles, rubbing them sensually using both hands. Then, pull back his foreskin and thoroughly wash and rinse his penis. A real turn-on for most men is for the woman to lean over the bath and take his penis into her mouth for a couple of seconds.

Use a warm towel to dry him thoroughly and lead him by the hand to the bedroom.

MASSAGE

Set the lights dimly and lie your partner back on the bed, putting him on his front.

Use oil to massage him. Do his back first then turn him over to rub his chest and stomach. Massage his legs, paying loving attention to the tops of his thighs.

ORAL SEX

Most men find oral sex irresistible. Yet it can be equally romantic for the woman as well as she repeatedly brings her man to the verge of orgasm or if the man comes inside her mouth.

Many men like to know what is going to happen, so tell him in detail what you are going to do.

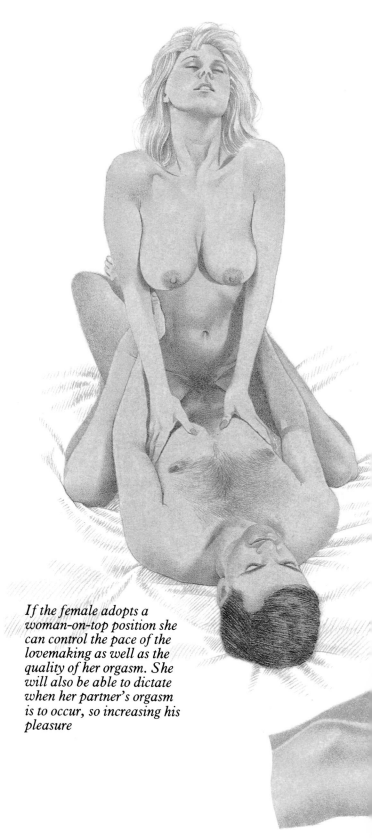

If the female adopts a woman-on-top position she can control the pace of the lovemaking as well as the quality of her orgasm. She will also be able to dictate when her partner's orgasm is to occur, so increasing his pleasure

Tell him that you are going to nibble his testicles and then lick along the underside of his penis before you take it into your mouth. Next, tell him either that you are going to suck him to the verge of orgasm or that he can come inside your mouth.

Position yourself comfortably so that he can see what you are doing to him – this is very erotic. Then alternate between just using your mouth and holding the root of his penis with your hand and sucking it with short, firm strokes.

POSITIONS

For the woman in control of lovemaking, the woman-on-top position where she faces towards her partner is the most romantic, both for him and for her. She is then free to kiss her partner and watch the effect her movements are having on him. She can then dictate the pace and vary the degree of penetration, to suit her and her partner.

Sit astride him and ease his penis inside you, supporting yourself with your hand behind his shoulders. Move slowly at first, up and down. Lean forward, allowing deep penetration, and nuzzle against his neck or kiss him full on the mouth. Then, switch your movements from side to side.

Increase the pace gradually. If your partner is nearing orgasm, do not hold back – allow him to come in his own time.

If your own orgasm is near, you can use your hand to massage your clitoris and increase the tempo until you both reach orgasm. Ease yourself away from him and nestle up to him.

Show your partner how much you desire him by taking the lead in lovemaking, but choose a position where you are facing him and are close enough to lean forward and kiss or caress him. To give your lover exquisite sensations, tighten your pelvic muscles as you slowly move up and down

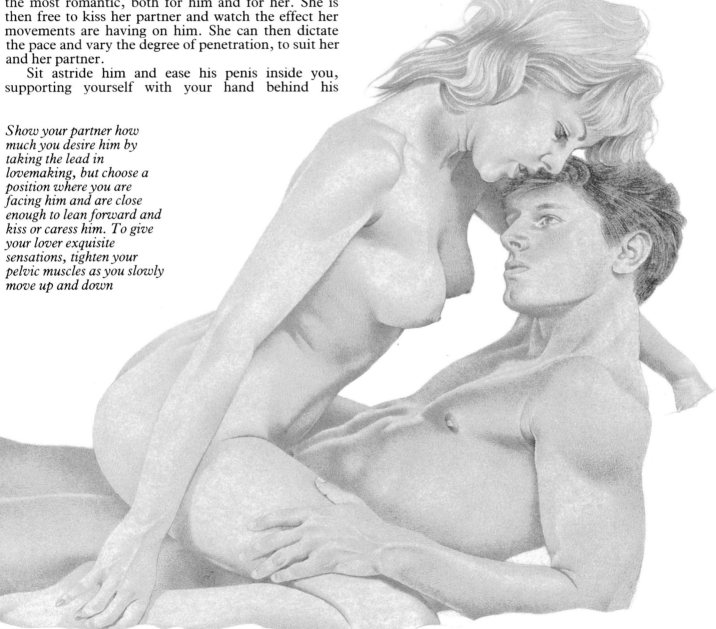

IMPROVING YOUR ORGASMS

The power of your orgasms will vary from time to time for many reasons, but if you feel you are missing out regularly, there are steps you can take to deal with this

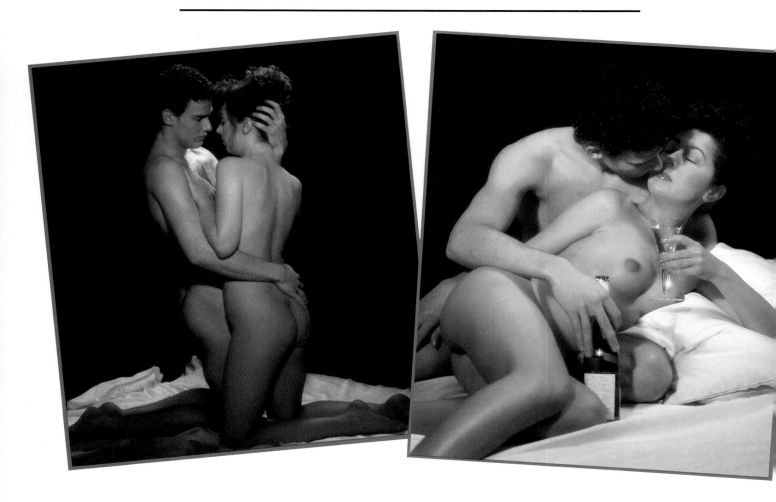

Although the vast majority of lovemaking and foreplay techniques concentrate – quite rightly – on unselfishness as a prerequisite for good sex, there will be times in most couples' lives when they will want to concentrate on the quality of their own orgasms and not just those of their partner. This does not mean that selfless lovemaking has to go out of the window, but it does demand, occasionally, a slightly different approach to sex from the person who wants to make lovemaking better for him – or herself. The ability to be honest with one's partner is the greatest aspect of a loving relationship.

WHY DO ORGASMS VARY
Most of us experience many thousands of orgasms in a lifetime. Yet, if we looked back on our love lives in old age, most of us would probably remember only a few episodes when our own orgasm was truly memorable. That is not to say that the others were not satisfactory, but some lovemaking episodes have a quality that sets them apart from all the others. Often there appears to be no reason, and it probably was not just the sex that made a particular memory linger on.

In fact, almost certainly, it would have been more to do with time and place and the feelings that the particular episode encouraged. For good orgasms are not just based on technique – masturbation can give us memorable orgasms as well.

For a man, there are biological reasons as well as emotional ones which explain these kinds of variation. Although the male sex organs are consistently efficient at creating seminal fluid – some younger men can make love many times during one session – if a man has not had sex for a period of time, the release of semen can be extraordinarily powerful. It is not just sexual frustration but a physiological need – a desire for sexual release.

A woman's sex drive varies much more subtly, both from woman to woman as well as during each

control and pace herself can both make a great deal of difference to the quality of, not just their own orgasms, but also those of their partner.

Combine that with the little tricks that lovers learn from each other and a continued desire to be inventive and to experiment sexually, and a couple's potential to increase the quality of their orgasms is immense.

FAMILIARITY
Many couples get locked into a fairly set and predictable approach to their own sexuality and that of their partner. A rigid routine of time and place followed by a predictable approach during every lovemaking episode can tire anyone's desire for sex.

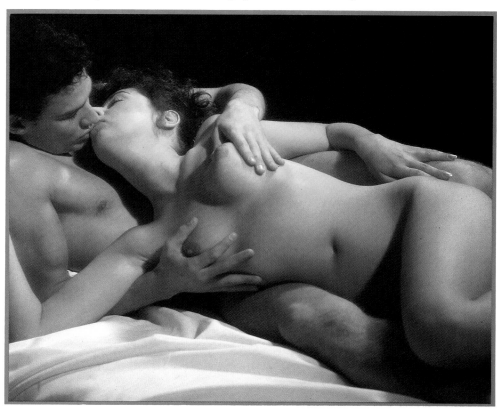

Making the most of your moments of lovemaking can help you both achieve memorable orgasms. Sharing those most intimate of moments and taking time to please each other, all add up to a deeper understanding of your partners' sexual needs. The more in tune your bodies are, the more you will know about bringing each other to orgasm

individual's own menstrual cycle. Add to that a generally more emotional approach to sex, where orgasm is part of a much more complete experience, and it becomes considerably more difficult to pin a woman's frustrations and sexual needs down.

Nonetheless, there will be periods in her life, in the same way as there are for a man, when her own orgasm is so powerful, so memorable, that she just longs to be able to repeat it more frequently.

SEXUAL TECHNIQUES
The most advanced techniques can leave both sexes cold if the mood is wrong, but in a loving relationship – or, at the very least, one where the physical attraction is still strong – the ability of a man to sustain and control his erection or the woman's ability to

What is worse is that the routines they are set in, however good, can all contribute to reducing the quality of the experience for the other. If, for example, kisses and caresses are always followed by oral sex and then penetration from exactly the same position, the experience can become quite forgettable.

Many couples could – if they were so inclined – put a stopwatch on their lovemaking and find that intercourse took place at the same time of the week, in the same place and that its duration varied by no more than a few seconds each time.

THE SOLUTION
The solution is obvious once the couple have realized the nature of their problem. After all, predictability in sex, by its very nature, does not happen overnight.

But if a couple do recognize that their own orgasms are less dramatic than they were and that they have lost that certain zest for orgasm that they used to have, the answer is quite straightforward. Some variation in their lovemaking routine is absolutely necessary.

Perhaps the order in which they approach sex might be reversed. Perhaps they could finish off with oral sex or try another position – or an existing one that they like from a slightly different angle. The time and the place could be changed – lovemaking on the settee in the living room, or on a rug in front of a fire can provide a remarkable change from the same time on the same night in bed.

In truth, because orgasm is as much a mental as well as physical experience, it is only really the mental approach that has to change.

IMPROVING YOUR PARTNER'S ORGASMS

It is important to realize, if you find that the quality of your own orgasm has deteriorated, that the same is probably true for your partner. If this has happened to you and you have been together for some time, the first step is to sit down and talk about it. If a couple can say truthfully and without embarrassment what they want – and what they would really like – the opportunities for experiment open up for both of them. Unfortunately, because it is so often easier to go for the simplest option, many couples never do get around to saying what they really want.

The advantage of doing this is that, once out in the open, it reveals a scenario for sex that so easily goes missing from many relationships. Sex between two loving partners can now become slightly illicit and adventurous – as it almost certainly once was in the early days of the relationship. And because the mind is the most powerful sex organ of all, if you know in advance that something exciting is going to happen between you at some point during the day, this becomes the first step to recreating exciting orgasms – not just for one of you – but for both.

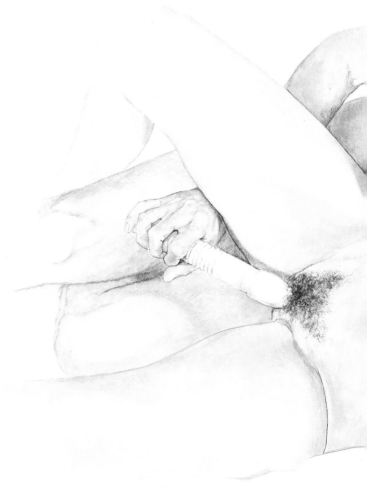

SOMETHING NEW

There are any number of techniques that a couple can use to improve the quality of their orgasms. But what follows are a series of suggestions that are slightly different in approach and which – unless of course the couple are already using them – can lend a degree of finesse and novelty to their lovemaking.

All the suggestions presume that you will both spend time in a certain amount of foreplay. If the ideas are already part of your sexual repertoire, this does not matter. You can always try them again or invent some slight variation to them that increases their novelty value.

The first two suggestions are directed at the woman who wants her partner to improve her orgasms for her. This is followed by two for the man who wants

the same thing. Finally, there are two ways in which a couple might try to improve their orgasms together.

FOR HER

A vibrator is one of the most popular ways in which a woman can achieve a novel sort of orgasm, either by using it herself or with her partner working it for her. The main purpose is to use it on the clitoris and, by increasing the speed, to bring the woman to orgasm as powerfully as possible. But a vibrator can lend itself to

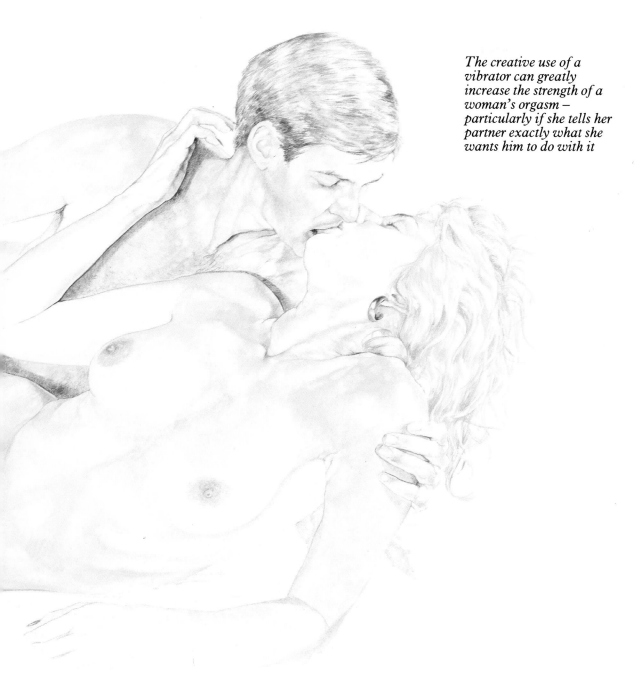

The creative use of a vibrator can greatly increase the strength of a woman's orgasm – particularly if she tells her partner exactly what she wants him to do with it

more creative use. You merely have to instruct your partner how you want it done.

You can lie down on the bed facing upwards or, alternatively, face downwards on the bed and place a couple of pillows under your stomach, as you would for a conventional rear-entry position.

Make sure that you are relaxed and tell your partner exactly what you want him to do. Be explicit so that there is no room for doubt. He is to concentrate solely on your orgasm – his own can always come later.

These suggestions assume that you have chosen to lie face downwards. Start off by parting your legs and raise your buttocks as high as possible. Get your

partner to start the vibrator at its lowest setting and begin using it to delicately massage your perineum. As you become more aroused, tell him to move on to your vaginal lips but without touching your clitoris yet. There is no need to hurry.

Then, when you feel that you are ready, get him to move on to your clitoris, increasing the speed setting a little. Do not let him move the vibrator around too much, just let it work almost on its own. Now, position yourself so that he can use his mouth and tongue on your clitoris instead and tell him to insert the vibrator into your vagina. Have him increase the speed setting and aim to use it as he would his penis,

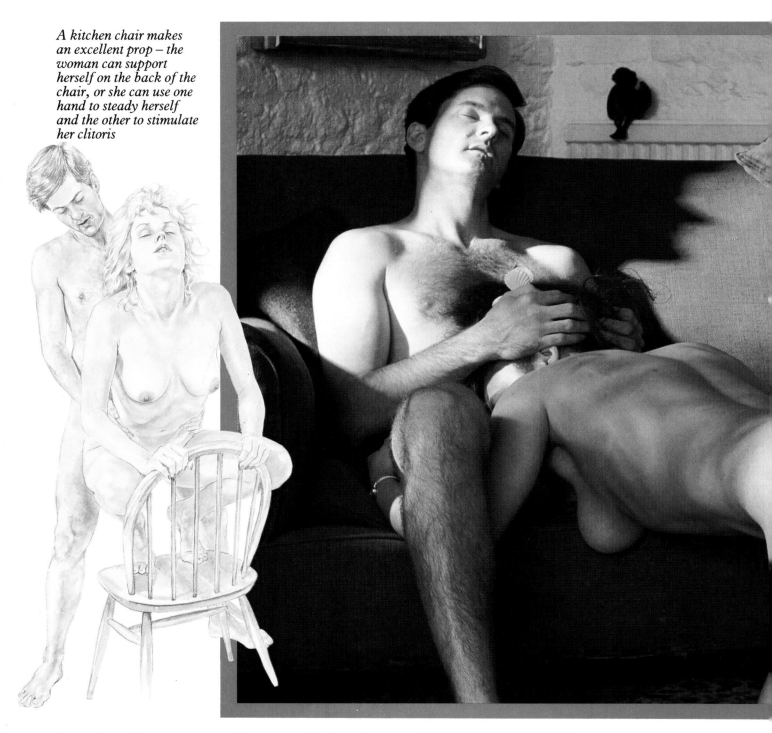

A kitchen chair makes an excellent prop – the woman can support herself on the back of the chair, or she can use one hand to steady herself and the other to stimulate her clitoris

increasing the pressure and tempo all the time. Encourage him to be as creative as he can and get him to keep the movements of his lips and tongue at much the same kind of tempo as the vibrator.

Alternatively, he can keep the vibrator working on your clitoris with a slightly increased speed setting and insert a couple of fingers into your vagina and mimic the movements of his penis in this way. He should be guided by your needs at all times. If you want him to abandon this at any stage and make love to you in this position, tell him what will please you most.

TAKING CONTROL

Sometimes, it is a good idea in a relationship for the woman to forget about her man's sexual needs and concentrate exclusively on her own. She can, of course, masturbate but she can also 'use' him to bring herself to orgasm. For a woman who is worried about adopting such a 'selfish' approach to lovemaking, it should help to realize that research has shown that most men do not mind at all being 'used' in this way – in fact, many relish it. And the woman can always

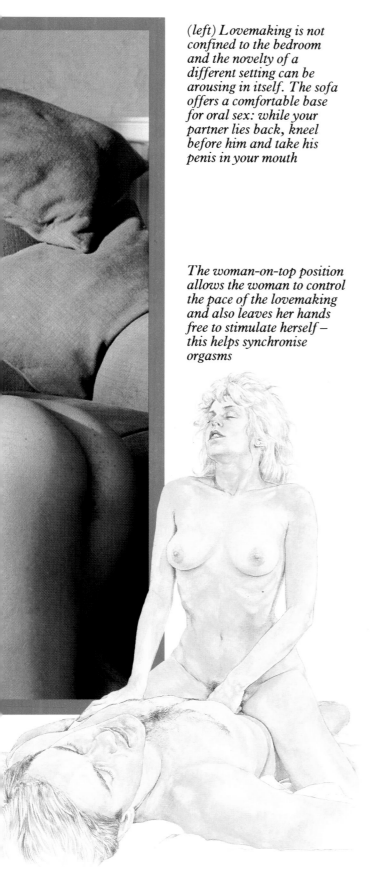

(left) Lovemaking is not confined to the bedroom and the novelty of a different setting can be arousing in itself. The sofa offers a comfortable base for oral sex: while your partner lies back, kneel before him and take his penis in your mouth

The woman-on-top position allows the woman to control the pace of the lovemaking and also leaves her hands free to stimulate herself – this helps synchronise orgasms

bring the man to orgasm later in some other way if this is necessary.

A good way of abandoning yourself in this way is to use one of the woman-on-top positions – if you want him to hit your G spot as he thrusts, then facing him is best – so that you are able to caress your clitoris yourself. By so doing, you will control the point at which you have your orgasm and, if you have G-spot-induced ones as well, you can ensure that your partner's penis hits the correct spot in your vagina in the way that you move your body.

The other advantage of this position is that it lends itself to a feeling of abandonment – particularly important if you want to control the pace of lovemaking.

Lay your partner back on the bed – or floor if you prefer. When he is erect, take his penis and insert it into your vagina. Start moving slowly at first and stroke your clitoris at the same time. Caress your breasts as well if you prefer. Take whatever approach you like – some women, for example, find this a particularly good position to use a vibrator on themselves as they 'use' their partner's penis in this way. Shift your buttocks until your partner's penis is hitting your G spot and try to direct your pelvis so that it hits it each time he thrusts. Increase the pace at which you are stimulating your clitoris and lose yourself as your orgasm approaches.

FOR HIM

There are any number of ways that you can encourage your partner to give you better orgasms. Most of them demand that she gives you what you especially like. Many of them will not involve her doing anything that – as a loving couple – you do not do sexually to each other anyway. It is just a slightly different approach.

It may be that you like her to dress for you in a particular way. Perhaps you want to be more passive in your lovemaking and her to take the lead. It may be that you want her to bring you solely to orgasm with her hands or mouth. Or there may be a favourite position that you would like to use – either in bed or somewhere different, such as in another room.

But for many men, an orgasm where their own G spot – their prostate gland – is stimulated can provide a very special sort of orgasm. This can be done in a number of ways but for a unique experience, it is best done either when your partner is fellating you or as you are having intercourse in a conventional way.

WITH ORAL SEX

Unless this is part of your usual lovemaking routine, you are going to need to tell your partner what you would like her to do. If it all seems a trifle selfish, do not worry. Explain that you will make it up to her another time, when you will concentrate entirely on her pleasure.

For comfort, she will need to have some KY jelly or oil handy if she is to put a finger into your anus. Lie down so that you are both comfortable and get her to start stroking your perineum very lightly. They key to this sort of dual orgasm is timing – if it is done properly, then it will probably be one of the most explosive orgasms you have ever had.

As she strokes you perineum, get her to start licking the tip of your penis as she would if she were fellating you in the usual way. Then, as she uses her lips and mouth on your testicles and runs her tongue up and down the shaft of your penis, she should take your penis into her mouth and start to gently suck on it.

As the pace increases and you become more aroused, she can put her finger into your anus and find your prostrate gland. You will need to adjust your position – probably bringing your knees up so that she can do this. When she finds it, she should then start to massage it, lightly, but insistently. As she brings you to orgasm with her mouth, you should find the dual sensations quite exquisite.

WHILE MAKING LOVE

The preparations here are the same – make sure that she has some KY jelly or something similar at hand and take up a missionary position, but with you kneeling and her pelvis raised towards you. This is to give her ease of access to your anus.

(above) Positioning yourself above your partner, rub your vulva and clitoris over his genitals to stimulate yourself to the point of orgasm before bringing his penis inside you

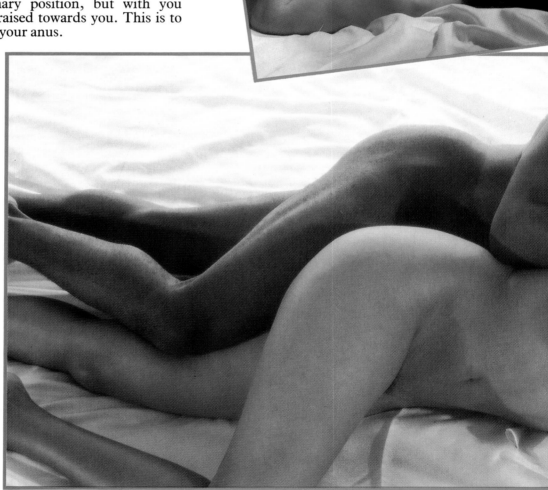

(right) Entering your partner from the rear while lying down can be particularly satisfying because of the closeness it allows couples. You can gently caress your partner's whole body while penetrating her from behind

As you make love to her, she should pop her finger inside you and start to gently massage your prostate.

FOR BOTH

One disadvantage of the above suggestions is that they tend to be one-sided. But there are a number of positions and techniques that provide something a little different. Some merely involve using positions that you have tried and tested before and just adding props that you find around the house.

REAR ENTRY
In fact, any household piece of furniture can act as a prop for lovemaking. The settee, the kitchen table or a household chair can all provide support for the woman and lend a lovemaking episode that extra something that may be missing in the bedroom.

Some couples find that an ordinary household chair can provide one of the simplest and most exciting options for them, either for quickie sex or after they have spent some time arousing each other.

Make sure that the chair is reasonably secure, though – a good idea is to place it against a wall to provide extra support and comfort.

The woman should use either the top of the chair

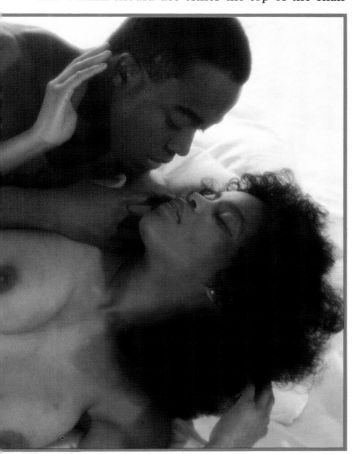

or the seat to place her hands so that her buttocks are offered invitingly to her partner. Then, it is simply a question of the man taking her from behind. She should use one hand to support herself and perhaps leave the other free to caress her clitoris.

ALTERNATIVES TO INTERCOURSE

Another way to orgasm – without involving intercourse but which puts a slightly different slant on orgasm – is for one partner to masturbate themselves to orgasm while using oral sex on their partner.

FOR HER

For the man, using his tongue and mouth on his partner while he brings himself to orgasm can be both unique and erotic. And for the woman, it can also be unusually arousing as she feels the sensations of his tongue and mouth on her as she watches him bring himself to orgasm.

Probably the best position for this is for the woman to sit astride his face – using her vaginal lips to give him a full genital kiss. In this way, she can 'use' his mouth to bring her to orgasm by controlling the movements of her lower body and increasing or decreasing the pace as she requires.

The man simply encircles his penis in his hands and masturbates the way he likes best. He should be able to sense when his partner's orgasm is coming and time his own to coincide with hers.

FOR HIM

The reverse – where the woman takes her partner's penis into her mouth and brings herself to orgasm by hand – can be equally pleasurable for both partners. Many men find the sight and sensations of the woman they love fellating them while masturbating both flattering and erotic.

The couple should take up a position that is comfortable. They can either lie down or make intelligent use of pillows so that the woman is sitting up. The man will probably enjoy the experience most if he is kneeling. A couple can easily experiment to see what they like best.

The woman then takes the man's penis into her mouth and starts to fellate him while masturbating in the way she likes best. If she senses that her partner is coming too soon, she can slow down the tempo with her mouth and increase the pressure with her hand and vice versa.

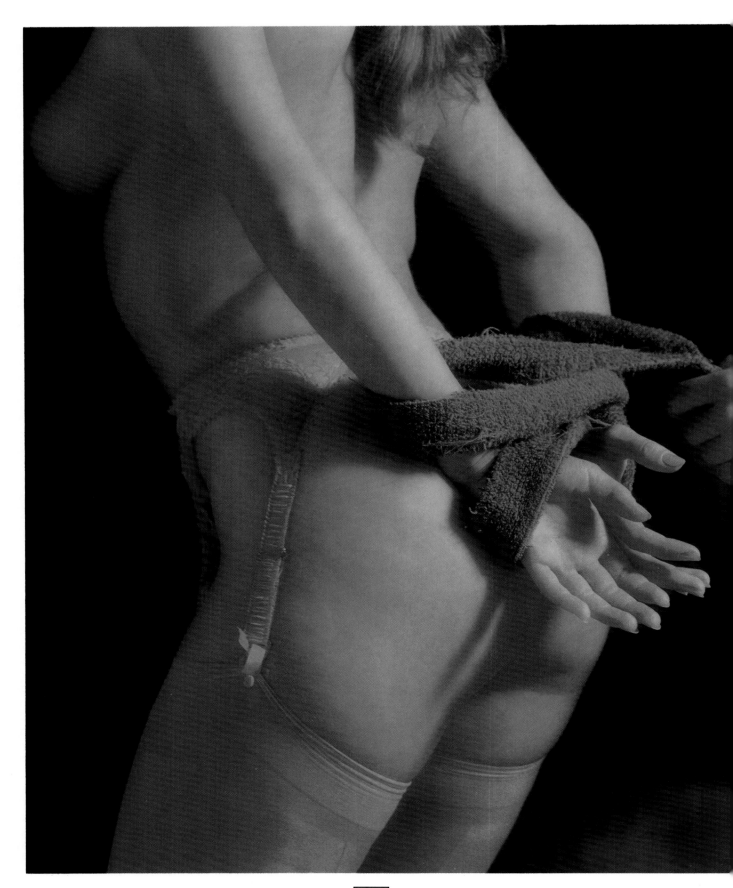

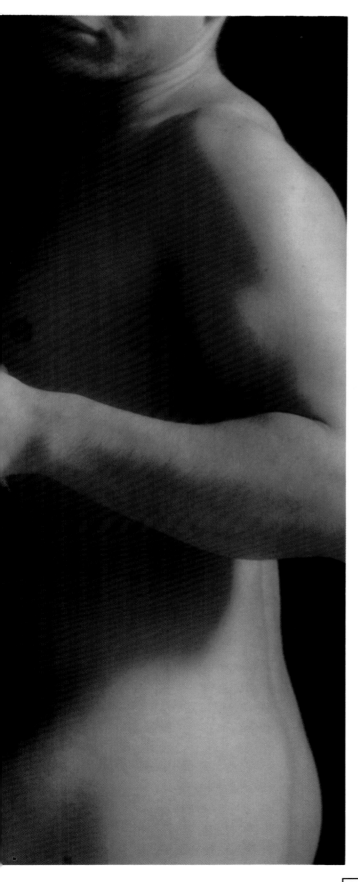

A DASH OF SPICE

Even the most successful sexual relationships can go through comparatively unexciting phases. With open minds and lively imaginations, you can put the sparkle back into your sex life, and reap the rewards of renewed closeness and contentment. Use these suggestions as a starting point, and let your own preferences and fantasies take over from there . . .

SEX AIDS

Considering that most people can function sexually with the body they were born with, the popularity of sex aids is perhaps surprising. However, many couples add fun to their sex lives by using sex toys

Sex aids and sex toys have an ancient history. Some of the best come from the East and for the most part the early ones have never been improved on. Given the technological age we live in, it is somewhat surprising that sex aids and toys have not progressed more than they have.

VIBRATORS
By far the most popular of all sex aids which sell by the million every year are vibrators. These are generally penis-shaped objects, although chemists' shops sell other sorts of 'massagers' which are often used in much the same way as the sex shop varieties.

Vibrators come in two main forms – battery operated and mains powered. Battery-driven ones have the advantage that they can be taken anywhere, but the mains versions are better because the quality of vibration remains constant.

As batteries run down, the power and quality of vibration diminishes and a vibrator loses much of its value. Given the price of batteries, many people leave them too long before replacing them and then complain that the vibration is poor.

Vibrators come in all sizes from small 10cm (4in) plastic ones that fit easily into a woman's handbag to giant 25cm (10in), or larger, versions covered in latex. The majority have a variable speed setting.

THE BASIC MODEL
The simplest vibrator, and arguably still the best, is a plastic phallic-shaped one. Its vibration is excellent but, as with almost all models, it is noisy, hard and cold. Those covered with latex are less noisy, less cold and more realistic – but are also more expensive.

It is possible, however, to put sheaths on vibrators to alter the nature of the stimulation when they are used vaginally. Various other attachments are available, but overall most women use their vibrator 'straight' and use it mainly on their vulval area.

DILDOES
These are highly realistic penis-shaped objects, made of latex-covered foam. They come in a variety of different lengths and thicknesses and some are fitted with a vibrator mechanism. Dildoes are usually available in black or skin colours. As an extra feature, some have a bulb on the end which, when squeezed, can squirt fluid in an imitation of male ejaculation.

Some women are turned on by the idea of a really large dildo inside them, but it tends to be more in their minds that in practice. Most women prefer using ones which are more 'realistic' in size, and so although some men buy larger dildoes as sex toys for their women, they are rarely used. One of the largest manufacturers makes dildoes sized from 0 to 6, and the size that sells best and appears to be the most popular is the second size up.

MALE MASTURBATION AIDS
Sex aids sold for men usually take the form of some sort of latex, hollow tube into which the penis is inserted. Some have a vibrator built in and others are inflatable to give a snug fit to the penis when erect. The most sophisticated type is an inflatable torso with a fairly realistic vagina in it.

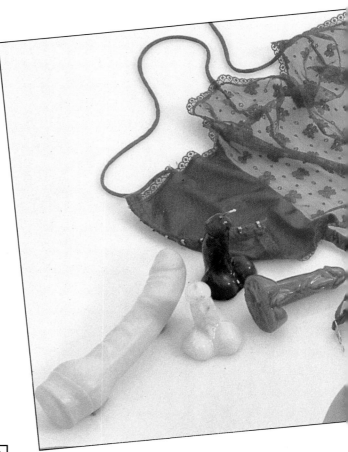

All of these prosthetics can be used by men who have no partner or whose partner is temporarily indisposed, for example after a gynaecological operation.

LOVE DOLLS
There are two basic types of love dolls. The first are simply plastic heads with gaping mouths into which a man can put his penis. Because they are made of plastic they are fairly fragile. The second are the better-known inflatable dolls.

Blow-up dolls are meant to be somewhat lifelike and the most sophisticated and expensive models have an open mouth, anus and vagina, all of which are designed to be penetrated. They are available with real hair, firm large breasts, erect nipples, pubic hair and an adjustable vagina, and can be easily cleaned.

Given the very high price – often in excess of £200 in the United Kingdom – it is difficult to know who exactly buys such dolls, but they certainly do sell.

ANAL STIMULATORS
Many men and women find that they enjoy anal stimulation – and some men are especially aroused by it. The simplest of stimulators are latex attachments to ordinary vibrators but there are also latex and plastic stimulators that are designed to be used anally. They are quite safe. Some have a vibrating mechanism, others do not.

Large, latex butt plugs are also available. They tend to be bought by people who enjoy having their anus widely stretched as a form of sexual arousal.

An anal stimulator with a very ancient history is Thai beads. The modern version of this consists of a thick plastic 'string' on to which are welded three medium-sized plastic balls. The whole thing is inserted into the anus and then, at critical moments, is pulled out of the anus to produce pleasant sensations.

SEX LUBRICANTS
Many couples find that there are certain times of the month when a woman's natural lubrication is low. When this is the case, a lubricant can make all the difference to the use of a vibrator whether on the vulva or in the vagina.

Dildoes really need lubricating every time they are used unless the woman is lubricating profusely herself. The latex has no innate slippery quality unlike the smooth, plastic surface of an ordinary vibrator.

Undoubtedly the best-known of all sex lubricants is KY jelly. It is, however, cold to use and has probably now been superseded by a new generation of more mucus-like lubricants, which offer a greater deal of 'realism'. Foremost of these in the United Kingdom is called Senselle. Versions of the same brand are available in other countries. There is a wide range of different lubricants on sale in sex shops, but they are generally more expensive and not nearly as good as KY jelly or Senselle.

SHEATHS
Almost all sex shops and catalogues offer a range of sheaths. They come in different colours and textures to give the woman added stimulation. There are so

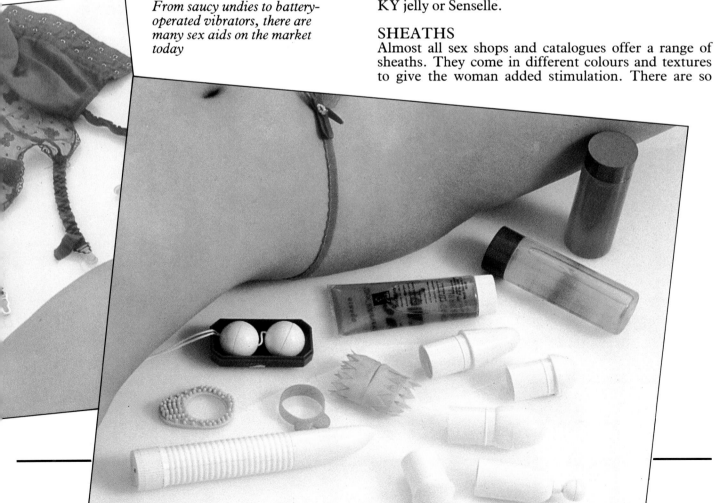

From saucy undies to battery-operated vibrators, there are many sex aids on the market today

many to choose from that it is a question of experimenting to discover which one works best for you. Many women find that textured sheaths do not enhance their vaginal pleasure at all, however.

PENILE TOYS

Given that so many men think their penis is inadequate it is hardly surprising that a vast array of sex aids and toys cater for this section of the market. Penile rings are probably the simplest of the options. These can be put around the base of the penis and prevent blood from flowing back into the body's circulatory system. Consequently, they produce a rock-hard erection with the penile veins standing out like blue cords.

Some couples enjoy the prolonged erection and such a device can be a real help to the man who would otherwise not have much of an erection or be able to maintain it for long enough.

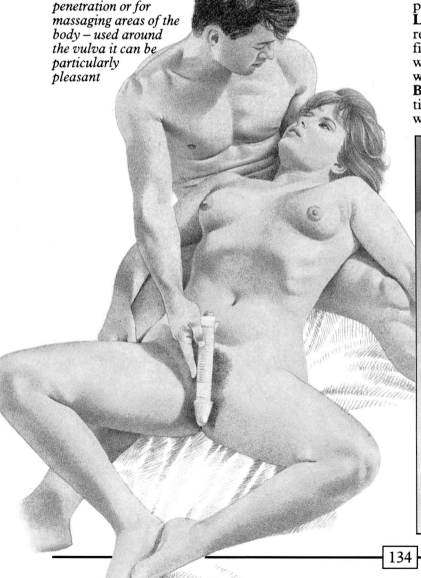

A vibrator can be used either for penetration or for massaging areas of the body – used around the vulva it can be particularly pleasant

The second most popular of the penile aids are the thick condom-like shapes that go over the penis and provide it with an extension of about 3.5cm (1½in). These can be useful for the woman who likes deeper penetration than her partner can manage, or for the man who thinks his penis is too short.

Most sophisticated of all are the penile enlargers. These are tubes that can have a vacuum suction applied to them and, placed over the penis, they do appear to enlarge it for a while. But more to the point, the enlargers can give a man the confidence which enables him to have a bigger erection.

The fact is that there is no known way of permanently effecting an enlargement of the penis once a man is past his full growth at about the age of 20.

CREAMS, SPRAYS AND POTIONS

Although there are many creams and potions on the market, none is of much value except, perhaps, in that they turn the man on by suggestions and so might just increase his ardour. 'Passion pills', various aphrodisiacs, ginseng and so on are all claimed to make a man more potent, but there is no clinical evidence that this is so.

Local anaesthetic creams or sprays can be valuable to reduce the sensitivity of the penis tip in those men who find that they ejaculate at the slightest stimulation within the vagina. The creams can also be used by men who simply want their erection to last longer.

Bust enlargement creams are almost certainly ineffective, although any cream lovingly massaged into a woman's breasts by her partner will enlarge them

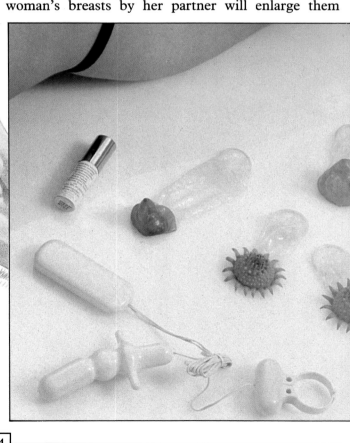

temporarily by arousal, possibly for several hours. **Pheromone sprays** have been tried by men who want to increase their allure to their woman. These aim to mimic a person's natural sexual odour, but research is confused as to how effective they are – for either sex.

Various creams are available that cause a mild irritation of the genital area to which they are applied. Some coupled find this adds to their pleasure but personalized foreplay is probably much more valuable – and cheaper.

SEXY UNDERWEAR
Most men, and quite a lot of women are turned on by sexy undies. These can be obtained by mail order from numerous outlets, including advertisements in very reputable magazines. Most outlets have inexpensive catalogues listing their wares.

Couples vary greatly in their tastes in this, as in all other sex aids and toys. Some go for blatant, tarty outfits, and others for classy, virginal underwear bought at expensive shops. If they enhance sexual pleasure they have served their purpose.

Although most women get their best sexual pleasure from their partner's penis or fingers, some enjoy other forms of vaginal stimulation. Vibrators and dildoes are the most popular but there are other possibilities too.

Latex finger covers can be put on the man's fingers before he stimulates the vagina. A plastic vibrating egg about 3.5cm (1½in) across can be very pleasurable for some women and an old trick exported from China is a pair of hollow balls each containing a heavy ball bearing. The woman or her partner inserts the balls into her vagina where they remain as she goes about her daily business. The ball bearings move in the spheres and stimulate the vagina. The balls are linked to one another and to a cord so that once in the vagina they can be easily removed.

CLITORAL STIMULATORS
These are latex attachments to penile rings which, when fitted around the base of the penis, come into contact with the woman's clitoral area to give her more stimulation during penetration. Some women find them useful, but many think they are annoying or irritating. It is very much a matter of personal taste.

BOOKS AND VIDEOS
Almost all couples have at some time or another used a sexy magazine or book to enhance their lovemaking. Erotic books have a very long history and today there are plenty of erotic and soft-core pornographic material to choose from.

Blue videos can be very arousing and can be valuable as mood setters. Sexy audiotapes are increasingly popular, too, and are good if you are turned on by what you hear rather than what you see.

TOYS AND FUN OBJECTS
Sex toys range from silly underwear to phallic candles, naughty playing cards to arousing zodiac charts. They raise a laugh, perhaps on a special occasion such as a birthday or wedding anniversary, and sometimes loosen inhibitions. They have little other value but, given that some couples take sex seriously and rarely get much fun out of it, perhaps even these have their place from time to time.

Sex aids can be fun, can be invaluable in enhancing a flagging sex life and can actually increase sexual pleasure in certain cases.

The choice is considerable and, with the right approach, the process of selection should be as enjoyable and interesting as it is stimulating for you and your partner.

Condoms come in all shapes, sizes and colours; some have unusual attachments designed for extra stimulation. If the idea of visiting a sex shop is embarrassing many companies can provide a catalogue of their aids

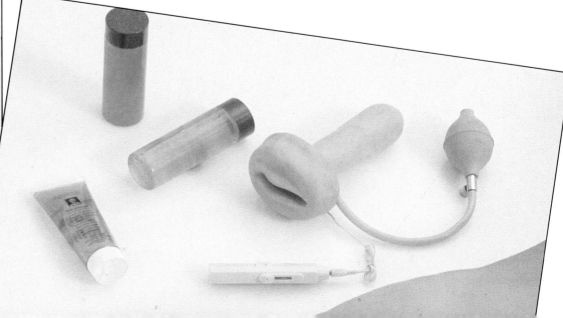

USING SEX AIDS

Many couples find that they can add a touch of excitement and variety to their sex life by using sex aids and toys. Most of these are perfectly safe, provided that they are used for the purpose for which they were designed. You are certainly more likely to come to grief if you use something that is not designed for this purpose.

The vast majority of aids need no more servicing other than a thorough clean, and if used with imagination in a loving relationship they can give countless hours of sensual pleasure.

VIBRATORS

If you are using a vibrator on your body – on the nipples, for example – then lubrication will not be necessary. But some women enjoy first oiling the part to be massaged with the vibrator. Try it with and without lubrication and see what you prefer. If you do not want to get oily, use talcum powder.

Be inventive and explore all over your body with the vibrator. You will probably be in for some surprises as you find all kinds of areas that feel terrific when vibrated and massaged. As you explore, try different speeds of vibration. Some areas of the body are stimulated most when the vibration is coarse and some when it is fine. Almost all vibrators have a speed adjustment for this purpose.

EXPLORING YOUR GENITALS

Once you have experimented with the vibrator on various parts of your body, you can now turn to your vulva. Start with the vibrator at a medium speed and rub it around the tops of your thighs and then move around the pubic area.

Next, stimulate the area between the vagina and anus. This part can be particularly sensitive on some women. Now open the lips of your vulva with the fingers of one hand and gently find where the vibrator produces the most arousing sensations.

Most women find that stimulating the clitoris directly is too powerful, or can actually be unpleasant, so start by experimenting around the clitoral area.

Whether you move the vibrator, or just put it in one spot and keep it there, is up to you.

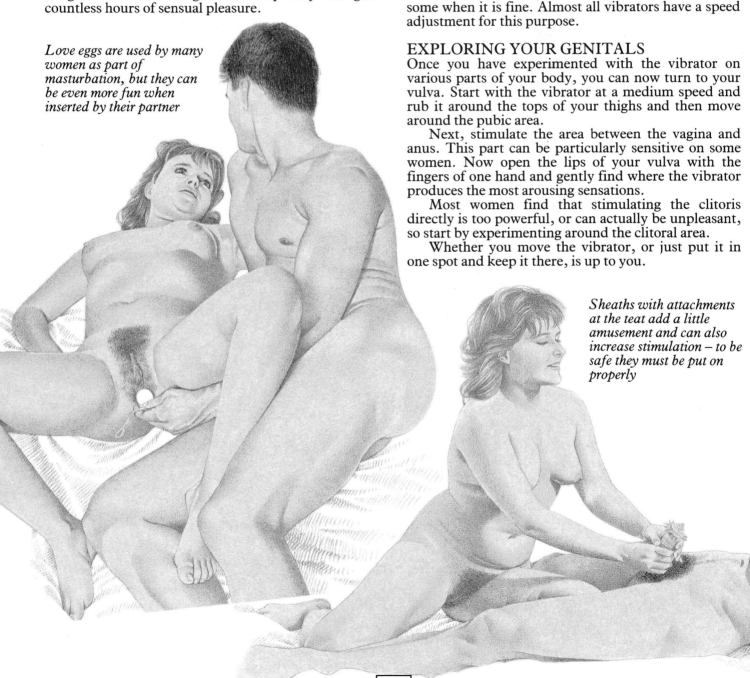

Love eggs are used by many women as part of masturbation, but they can be even more fun when inserted by their partner

Sheaths with attachments at the teat add a little amusement and can also increase stimulation – to be safe they must be put on properly

After a few minutes' experimenting, you will have a fairly good idea of what you most enjoy. If you start to have really powerful sensations you might want to go straight on to have an orgasm. If you prefer not at this stage, try the vibrator inside your vagina.

By now you will probably be highly aroused and so will be wet with natural secretions. If not, use a little saliva on the vibrator, some KY jelly or one of the new types of sexual lubricant such as Senselle. Gently insert the vibrator into the vagina until you begin to experience pleasurable sensations.

Many women receive very little or no sensation from this, but there are other things you can try such as vibrating the entrance to the vagina, vibrating deep inside all around the cervix, stimulating the G spot on the front wall of the vagina and using the object to produce penis-like thrusting movements with or without the vibration unit switched on.

Lastly, you can try playing with the vibrator around the anal region. Many women enjoy the sensations produced by vibrating this area and a few, especially those who enjoy anal sex, like the vibrator actually inside them.

MEN AND VIBRATORS
Men can enjoy being stimulated with a vibrator, but they rarely get as much pleasure out of it as their partner. Some men like certain parts of their body stimulated and a few like their genitals vibrated but it rarely causes an orgasm as in women, at least not without other, manual or oral, caresses too.

A man whose anus is extremely sensitive can greatly enjoy both external and internal vibration and, as in women, the G spot (prostate gland) can be stimulated to great effect with a vibrator. This can best be done with the man lying down with his legs pulled back and the vibrator inserted several inches and aimed at the front wall of the back passage.

IMPROVING ORGASM
Perhaps the most important use of vibrators is for women who are unable to have orgasms without powerful stimulation from a source other than their fingers. These women can usually learn how to have an orgasm with a vibrator and then transfer the ability to their own, or their lover's, fingers.

Many women are concerned that they will become addicted to the strong stimulus of a vibrator and then be unable to do without it, but this is rarely the case.

DILDOES
A dildo is easy to use and, unlike a real penis, has great stamina so is ideal for the woman who needs a lot of thrusting in order to have an orgasm. Most women when they masturbate insert two fingers into their vagina so a dildo that stimulates this kind of size is probably best.

It can be held still, thrust in and out just inside the vaginal entrance, or thrust deeply in and out as the woman likes. All three can be pleasant and arousing even when incorporated within one orgasmic cycle.

Apart from keeping them clean and ensuring that they are well lubricated there are no particular problems in use.

More unusual dildoes have a squeezable bulb at the end you can hold which can be made to ejaculate milk

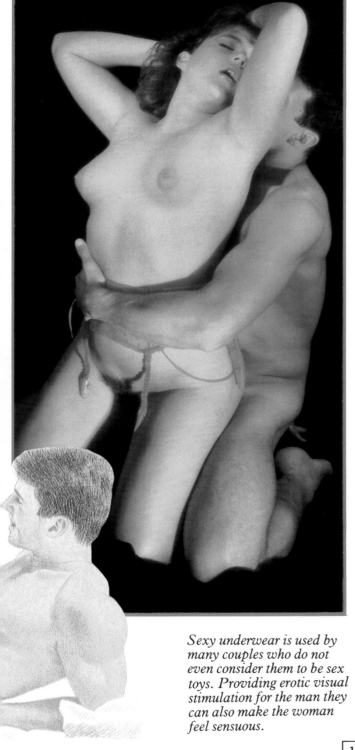

Sexy underwear is used by many couples who do not even consider them to be sex toys. Providing erotic visual stimulation for the man they can also make the woman feel sensuous.

or water as the woman climaxes. Double-ended dildoes are suitable for two women at once, and yet others can be inflated by squeezing a bulb so that the girth of the device can be altered to fit the vagina of the user. This is useful for the woman whose vagina has become slack after having more than one child.

SHEATHS
Textured and contoured sheaths can be obtained in a variety of sizes and shapes. They all give a slightly different vaginal sensation when used on a man's penis or on a vibrator. Just how useful they are is difficult to say, because many women get little or no sexual pleasure from them.

When using them on a penis they must be donned in the same way as an ordinary contraceptive sheath. Extra care should be taken, though, because with their novelty element, it is easy to forget that contraceptive precautions are still important and that they must till be effective as well as increasing stimulation and providing a bit of fun.

Some sheaths are washable and so can be re-used, but make sure which these are or you could run the risk of an unwanted pregnancy.

SEXY UNDERWEAR
These are, arguably, the most widespread of sex 'aids', and the ways in which they can be utilized are numerous, but here are a few tips:
☐ Make the giving and receiving of gifts of sexy undies into a game. Take the opportunity to dress up in them as soon as you can so that your man knows that you like them. Do a striptease for him, or let him undress you when you are wearing them for the first time. Arouse him by stripping very slowly.
☐ Leave at least one piece on when making love. For example, if the set consists of a bra, pants, suspender belt, garter and stockings, then leave the suspenders and stockings on to make love in. You will both find this highly arousing.
☐ If the man is away from home he can send some sexy undies through the post to his partner. She can then wear them while he is away and write or phone to tell him all about them. This can be highly exciting for some men.
☐ When you are going out somewhere special, leave off a part of your underwear.
☐ Pretend that the woman is a model for a catalogue and get her to pose in her sexy undies for photos. She can strip them off as the session progresses.

CLITORAL STIMULATORS
It is important to go easy when using one for the first time in case it irritates or annoys your partner. The kind of stimulation they apply is very non-specific, and most women have highly specific needs when it comes to stimulating their genitals.

Once the ring is in place, be careful not to thrust too hard as these stimulators do not have the elasticity of human skin. It is probably better to go for gently rotating and wriggling movements.

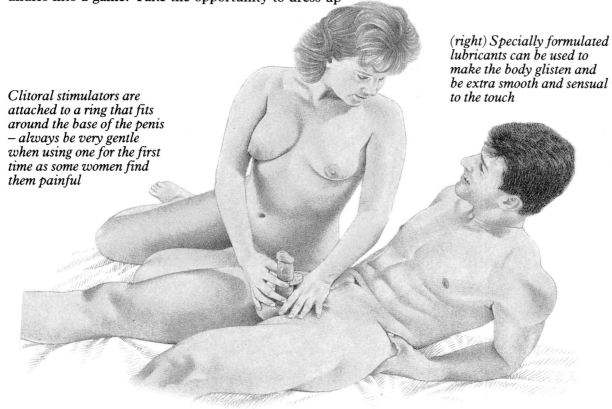

Clitoral stimulators are attached to a ring that fits around the base of the penis – always be very gentle when using one for the first time as some women find them painful

(right) Specially formulated lubricants can be used to make the body glisten and be extra smooth and sensual to the touch

PENILE RINGS

Penile rings are quite useful, but need to be chosen with considerable care. Too small a ring can be painful as the swelling penis find itself trapped and too large a ring will be ineffective.

Put the ring on well before penile stimulation starts or it could be difficult to get on at all. Once the man has ejaculated, he should wait until the penis has subsided a little before trying to remove it, as it could cause pain or even damage trying to get it off a semi-erect penis.

Only ever use rings that are specially made for the purpose. Never use a ring made of wood or metal because, should trouble occur, it can be almost impossible to remove and may even call for surgery.

The best type is a latex, or other rubber, ring that can easily and speedily be released if there are signs of trouble or the pressure of blood in the penis becomes too high, thus causing pain. The problem with rigid rings is that, even if the penis becomes painful because of its excess blood, nothing can be done to release the pressure until the penis subsides a little. This can take some time.

MALE MASTURBATION AIDS

These hollow latex tubes, with or without a vibrator mechanism, are straightforward to use. They simply need to be kept scrupulously clean and then well lubricated immediately prior to use. They are mainly used by men who have no partner, either permanently or temporarily, and certainly help give additional sensations to those obtained manually alone.

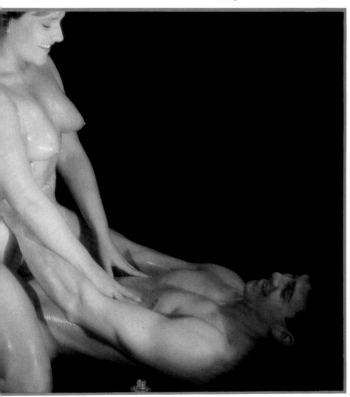

Sex dolls, whether in the form of heads or whole bodies, require similar care and maintenance, especially the dolls which, because they can be very expensive are well worth looking after.

ANAL STIMULATORS

The simplest of these are attachments to ordinary vibrators and are straightforward to use. As long as they are firmly attached to the vibrator and cannot possibly get lost, all should be well. They are very narrow and cannot do any harm to the anus itself.

When inserting anything else into the anus, be sure that you go gently and stretch the anal sphincter slowly or it can be very painful. Special butt plugs, wide latex aids, that stretch the anus considerably, are available. These are not dangerous provided they are not inserted too deeply and so could get lost. They also need to be inserted slowly so as not to damage the delicate tissues.

If ever anything you do to your anus makes it bleed, it is probably best to stop and not to do it again. Never put anything into the anus that is not made for it. The anal muscles can be very powerful and things can break off and become trapped inside.

SEXUAL LUBRICANTS

For most love-play, the best and most widely-available sexual lubricant is saliva. However, if you have any infection of the mouth or throat, cold sores around your lips or anything that gives you cause for concern, then do not use saliva, but a commercial lubricant such as KY jelly or Senselle. KY is an excellent all-purpose lubricant but feels cold straight from the tube, and is not all that realistic when compared with natural vaginal secretions. Senselle is a newer and more realistic lubricant, available in the United Kingdom, that feels just like vaginal secretions. It is odourless, taste-free and not cold.

Although saliva is fine for applying to the penis or vagina during foreplay and intercourse, many sex aids call for a lubricant that is more tenacious and does not dry up so quickly. Hence the need for commercial lubricants. Latex takes a lot to lubricate well and saliva rarely works effectively. Plenty of lubrication is essential if the vagina is not aroused and is always necessary in any form of anal activity.

VAGINAL STIMULATORS

There are no special tips for using these specially made toys and aids, but it is worth pointing out the dangers of other things that some women use in their vaginas.

Almost any penis-shaped object can be pleasant to masturbate with but many are fraught with danger. Nothing breakable should ever be put into the vagina.

A spherical object, like a small orange, may be highly stimulating to push into the vagina at climax but can be difficult, or even impossible, to remove without surgery. The vagina contracts down on such objects and because they are so slippery and round they are difficult to remove.

MAKING A
SEXY VIDEO

*For the loving couple, making an erotic video can be a stimulating
experience – allowing them both a new perspective on their sex life*

Making your own erotic video should be fun. Not only does it give you the chance to see yourselves making love, it also enables you both to direct and star in your own movie.

Much of the pleasure in making a video will be in the preparation. For professional movie makers, this is where the maximum effort goes so that time and expensive film are not wasted.

You will not take your erotic video quite so seriously, but attention to detail is required so that the actual filming runs reasonably smoothly. The more effort you put into the product, the better the end result will be.

TEST SHOTS
First, you both need to familiarize yourselves with the workings of the camera. You should be able to use it so that the perspective can be altered during the actual filming. Try firing off a few feet of video on test shots. It will not be wasted as you can always record over it again. You also need to practice to make sure that you get the focus and framing right.

These test shots will not only help you to become familiar with the workings of the camera, they will also help you overcome any camera shyness. So, while one of you handles the controls the other should be trying out positions, poses and actions. Some of these should include scenes where your back is turned to the camera. This should help you act more naturally.

ZOOMING
While one partner is doing this, the other can be practising various camera techniques, including zooming – moving the camera's view point either physically or optically into the scene – and panning – swinging the camera steadily across the scene.

TOGETHER ON SCREEN
Your erotic video is not going to be restricted to showing each partner in turn. You will need some

scenes at least when the two of you are on screen together, to develop the storyline further.

To achieve this, it is best that you have a tripod so that you have a full range of adjustments for the position of the camera. Alternatively, you will have to find a secure place to rest the camera, but this may limit your options.

Once you have set the camera up, feed its output direct to your TV set which you can use as a monitor. (On the camcorder type of camera – where the camera and video recorder are all in one – this may not be

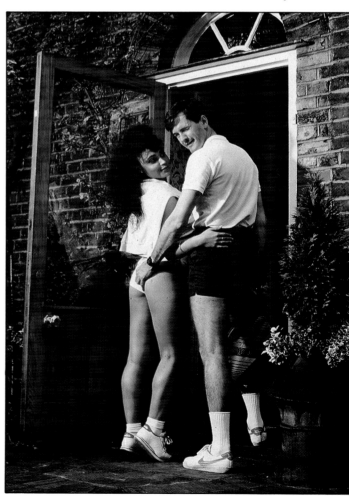

Try to have a natural start to the story – arriving home after a run or a game of tennis gives a good opportunity for both partners to be wearing skimpy clothes. Set the camera up so that you can get both players into at least some of the scenes

THE STORY BOARD

Professional film makers turn their scripts into a story board before proceeding with the shoot. The story is essentially translated into a cartoon strip with each scene and camera shot drawn out in detail.

This approach may not be necessary for a home video, but it does give you a chance to combine some of the striking images that you came across in your test shots with the main story line. Each scene can then progress to a narrative and visual climax.

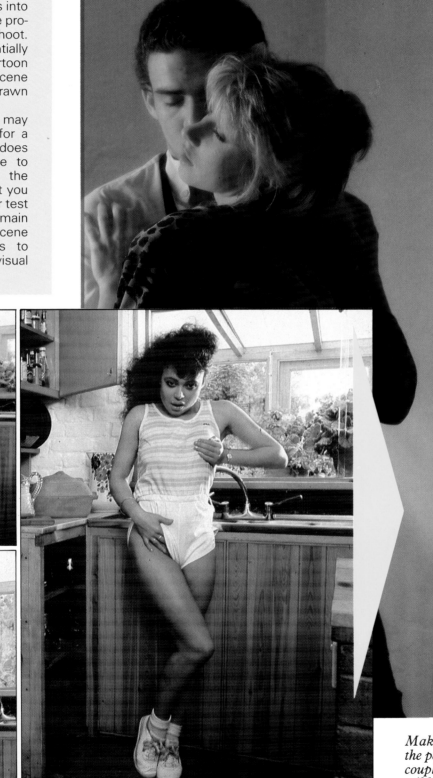

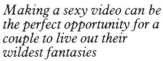

Making a sexy video can be the perfect opportunity for a couple to live out their wildest fantasies

possible and to see yourself you will have to shoot direct to tape.)

Next, place the camera well back, rehearse certain scenes and take up various positions with your partner without leaving the frame. This will require a little practice to frame the picture as well as possible.

After a time you will get a feel for it. Then you will find that you develop a sense for playing to the camera. You will be able to assume certain positions, knowing that they make pleasing images on screen, without having to glimpse over at the monitor, or check the tape, too often.

LOVE STORY

Although the image of two people making love on screen is in itself interesting, the appeal of the story is age-old. A video will have a more long-lasting appeal if it has a strong story-line.

It is best to write a short shooting script so that each of you knows what to do. This could include lines of dialogue, camera and stage directions. But do not make these too hard and fast, The script should leave certain areas open for improvization.

Coming up with ideas for stories should not be difficult. You may find it pleasing to re-live an event in your own life – such as the first time you made love.

Alternatively you could act out a scene from a favourite film.

LOCATION

It is probably best to avoid acting out certain fantasies on screen. These can often appear banal when played

THE CONTRACT

No movie star goes to work without a cast-iron contract. You and your partner must agree under what circumstances the video is to be shown and what happens to it if you split up at some point in the future.

It is best that you agree that only the two of you should be allowed to see the video and that it is destroyed if you separate.

You should find some place safe to keep it too, especially if you have children in the house.

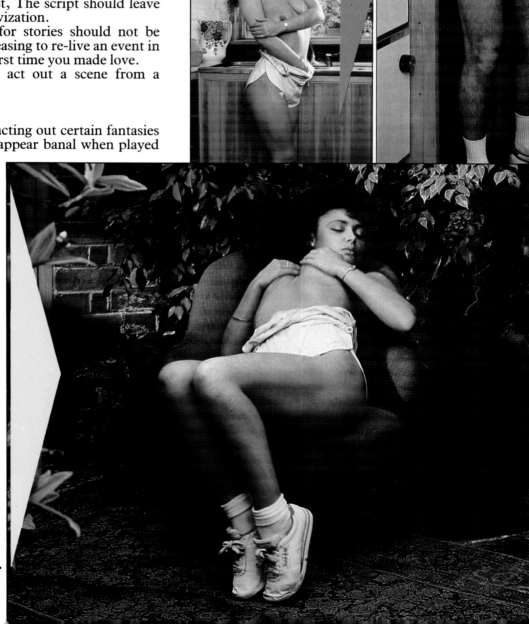

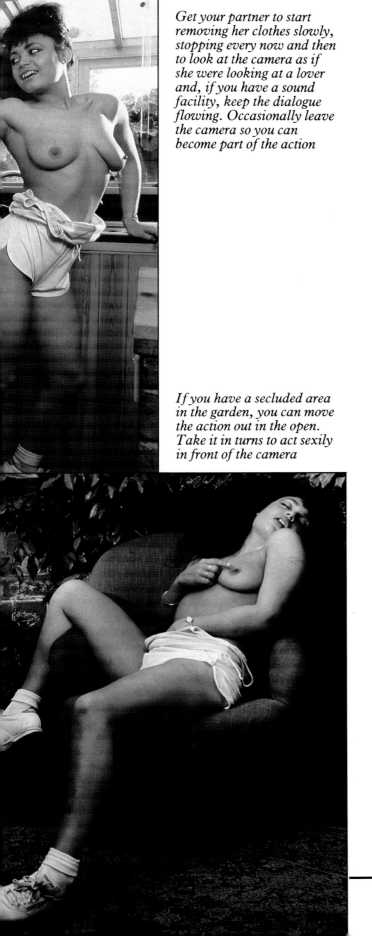

Get your partner to start removing her clothes slowly, stopping every now and then to look at the camera as if she were looking at a lover and, if you have a sound facility, keep the dialogue flowing. Occasionally leave the camera so you can become part of the action

If you have a secluded area in the garden, you can move the action out in the open. Take it in turns to act sexily in front of the camera

WORKING THE CAMERA

Modern video cameras are easy to use. Most have automatic focusing and many also have automatic exposure systems – with most cameras all you will have to do is select the colour temperature for natural or artificial light.

However, as most of your filming is likely to take place indoors in adverse light conditions, you will have to experiment with both the camera and the sort of artificial lighting that is most appropriate. Check that lighting conditions are suitable for filming each time you shoot.

The most important feature that is left to manual control is the zoom. This allows the point of view of the camera to move in and out of the picture. It is important that you use this facility steadily and smoothly. Some cameras have a motorized zoom which makes smooth operation much easier.

The camera's user manual will explain how to use the other controls. Familiarize yourself with it thoroughly, then try out the camera on more innocuous subjects – such as a day on the beach or a country picnic – before moving on to sexy videos.

out – as you will see if you have ever watched some of the poorer 'blue' movies.

Once you have an idea what is going to go on in your video, you need to decide on the location. Probably you will want to use your own house as you are going to need privacy. But you are not going to use the whole of the house and it is best to plan out which corners are going to suit the action.

Remember that if you are filming in a room, at most you can only show two of the walls at any one time. Pick the best two. But also be inventive. You may be able to take some interesting shots up and down the staircase and through windows and doors.

The camera need not always be at chest height either. Interesting shots can be achieved shooting upwards from the floor, or down from the ceiling – in awkward situations these shots can be faked by shooting the scene reflected in a strategically placed mirror. Be as creative as possible.

LIGHTING

Remember, too, that in the absence of any powerful and expensive artificial lighting you are going to have to rely on sunlight, so the room with the biggest windows is going to be the best. You will not want a room where you are overlooked, though, as you will not be able to draw the curtains under most circumstances without losing more light.

However, if you use a room that receives direct sunlight, on a sunny day you will have problems with the contrast between light and shade. In this case, you can soften the effect with a pair of lace curtains.

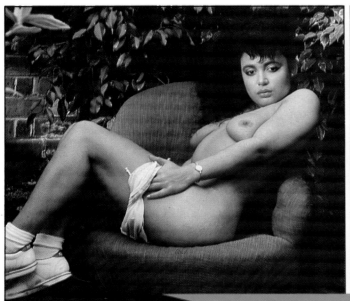

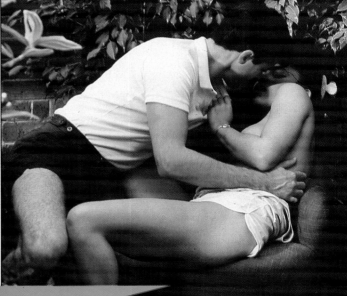

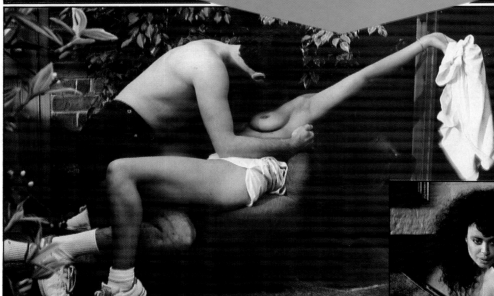

As the excitement builds up, the striptease should continue with more garments being divested. Now is the time to set the camera on the tripod and join in. Make sure you are both in the frame and avoid any movements which will lead you out of the picture

A secluded garden may afford other interesting possibilities. But the whole garden does not have to be secluded: if one corner is not overlooked, you may be able to stage the action there, in privacy, while the camera itself is set up in the more open part. Try out the possibilities with a stills camera in advance.

SHOOTING OUTDOORS

The more adventurous may plan to shoot some, or all, of their video out in the countryside or perhaps on a beach. If you do decide to do this, choose somewhere that you are sure is deserted as it is against the law to expose yourself or perform any 'indecent' act in a public place.

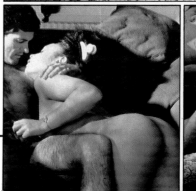

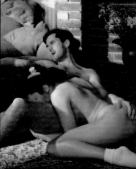

WARDROBE AND PROPS

Although clothes may seem superfluous to an erotic video, you may well decide to start out clothed and shed your garments during the filming. Remember that you will want to look erotic and alluring – or at least presentable – at each stage of undress. Men, especially, should remember to take their socks off before their trousers and underpants.

Although the temptation may be for the woman to wear stockings and suspenders, there are plenty of other erotic possibilities. If you are uncertain about what to wear, try looking through a catalogue of glamorous underwear for ideas.

Depending on the story line, you may need some special props for your film. Remember to organize these before the filming and put them in the right position before each scene. And if you want to reshoot a scene, remember to return them to their proper place.

BODY CARE

The most important prop in your erotic movie is going to be your own body.

Stay out of your clothes and avoid sitting down until you are ready for the first shot. You will not want the marks of tight clothing or a hard seat pressed deeply into your flesh to be captured on film.

Make up is optional, but it often helps. Women may find that they have to exaggerate their normal style to give the right impression on screen, while men may benefit from a little eye makeup. Bruises, and any other unsightly marks should be covered with foundation before any filming begins.

SHOOTING THE VIDEO

When the time comes to shoot the video, remember that, above all, the idea is to have fun. No matter how well you have planned the shooting something is bound to go wrong. But, the chances are that these 'out-takes' will be a memorable part of the film.

STICKING TO THE SCRIPT

Keep your shooting script handy throughout filming and try as far as possible to stick to it. But if something spontaneous and genuinely exciting occurs, capture the moment on tape while it is happening. It may be better than anything you had planned and if you stop and try to recapture that moment later you may find that it has been lost forever.

STRIPTEASE

The easiest scenario to film is a straightforward striptease – simply because one partner can handle the camera while the other supplies the action. But try and be inventive. Move the camera and alter the framing. Try striptease on the move, down a corridor or up or down the stairs.

If you can, move the camera around your partner and film them from all angles as they remove their clothes. The stripper can either be unconscious of the camera, as if they are simply undressing in the privacy of their own home, or they can be very seductive and play up to the camera as if they were stripping to turn on a lover. Remember – there are no fixed rules, because you are both director and co-star.

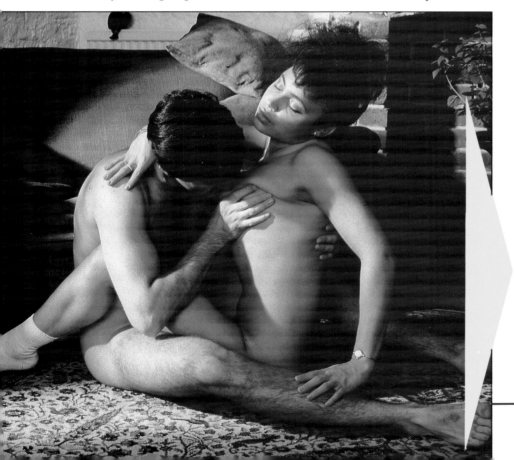

As the action progresses, move back indoors. Your partner can now remove the rest of her clothes, before she totally undresses you. For some couples, oral sex will be a feature of their lovemaking and it will certainly ensure that the man achieves a good erection

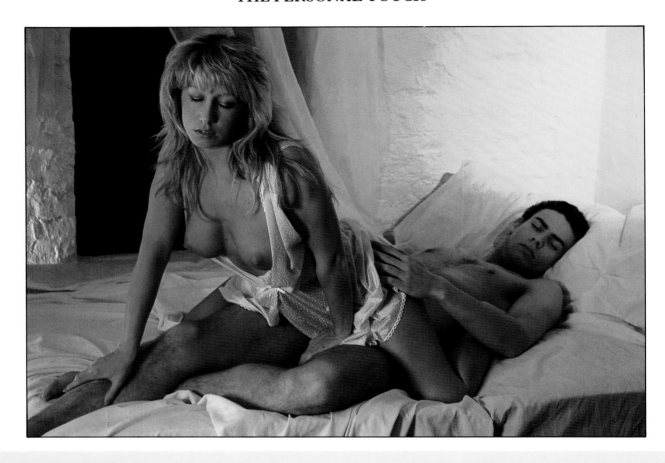

EDITING THE VIDEO

Much of your approach to showing a video must be governed by whether you have editing facilities or not. All you need to edit is two recorders. By recording sections of one tape on to another, you can cut out bits you do not want.

If you have a camcorder, you may be able to use that as one recorder and your domestic play-back machine as the other. Some camcorders, however, do not have a playback facility. If you have one of them, or a straightforward video camera, you can borrow or hire a second machine. That way, you will be able to shoot your script in any order that you like and then reorder it later. You will also be able to cut out unwanted sections. For 'arty' effects you can repeat sections and freeze frame.

(above) As you both approach your climax any inhibitions about being filmed will probably fade away

Finally, with the camera secure on its tripod, you can become totally involved in lovemaking, changing positions as the mood takes you to add a bit of variety. Do not forget to keep the dialogue flowing as you and your partner head towards orgasm.

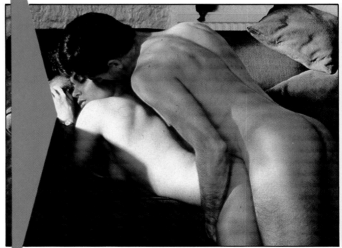

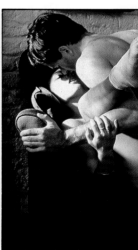

OTHER MOVEMENTS

A portable camera can also find a subject. It can come in through the bathroom door and find a naked man in the bath, look through a window to see a naked girl combing her hair. Often the quality of the light can lend such scenes a certain poignancy.

In scenes of masturbation the camera can zoom quickly in on to face, hands or genitals. If you have editing facilities you can cut between these quickly to good effect.

Panning slowly across a naked body, from head to toe – or from toe to head – can have a lingering eroticism, as can panning slowly across the scene to find a nude in a far corner. Try to incorporate shots which enhance any fantasy element of the storyline. Be bold – a lack of inhibition will make a better result.

ANTICIPATION

What is not seen is often more erotic than what is – such is the quality of the imagination.

If the camera follows the feet of a subject up the stairs while clothes are falling around them on the steps, the viewer will draw only one conclusion. They are going to see a naked body somewhere upstairs, possibly in bed, ready for lovemaking.

The anticipation can be heightened further by making figures disappear around doors or glimpsing a naked body for a fleeting moment in a mirror and the final video will be all the more erotic.

ACTION

If you do not have any editing facilities, you are going to be restricted when filming actual intercourse. Most video cameras do not have remote control facilities, although a straightforward video camera is activated by pressing 'record' on the player, which you may be able to place in a handy position – perhaps under the bed or behind a piece of furniture.

With a camcorder which has no playback facility, you will essentially be restricted to one static shot and you will have to devise your scene so that one of you has a reason to walk on to the set at the beginning – after switching on the camera – and off again at the end – to switch it off.

Only if you have two machines will you be able to edit these bits out.

VIEWING

The pleasure of a video is not just in the making of it – watching the results of your efforts should be just as much fun. You and your partner should watch the raw tape – the rushes – deciding which shots should be left in and which cut out, then edit the tape into shape.

Once you have the final version ready, you should make quite a thing of the first showing. Have a glass of wine, close the curtains and dim the lights, and watch your movie on a comfy sofa or in a bed. You may want to re-live some of the highlights and act out your fantasies – without the camera running.

The video should also show the time after orgasm, when the couple's delight in the experience of each other should be made apparent

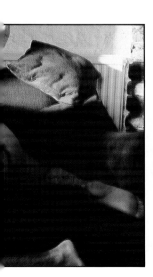

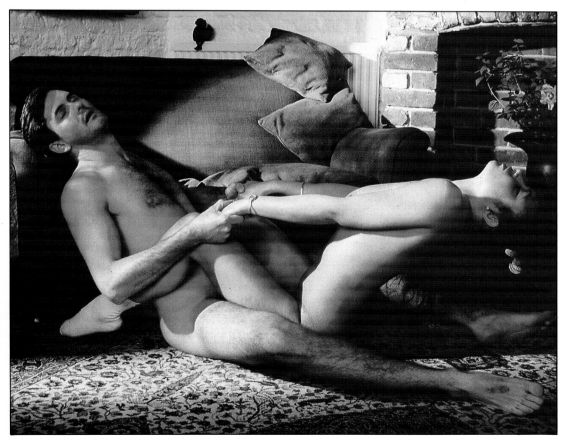

FETISHISM

Fantasy and fetishism are generally closely linked. But can a fetish ever be allowed free expression in a couple's relationship?

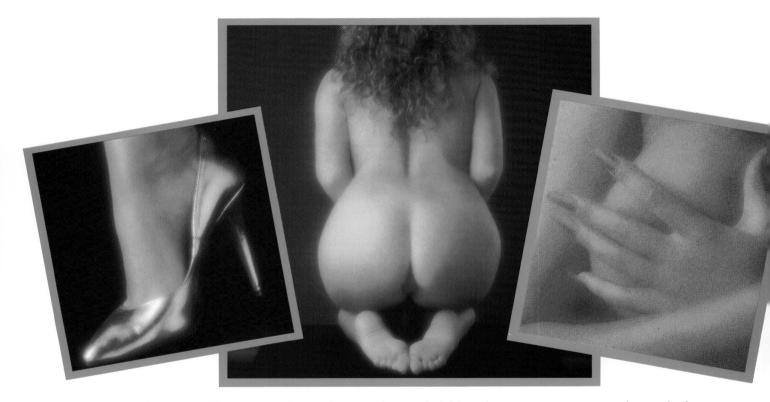

Most of us enjoy little 'extras' or enhancers in our sex lives, if only from time to time. These take many forms from sexy undies to sex toys, from unusual locations to new positions. Whatever we do, though, is usually of fleeting importance to us – it enhances that particular lovemaking episode, or perhaps a few occasions, but is not a compulsion that is specifically needed in order to make sex enjoyable.

WHAT IS A FETISH?
A fetish is usually a practice that is deeply ingrained in our psychosexuality. Those who have them – usually men – find that they have a craving or need for a particular object or part of a woman's body without which they simply cannot truly enjoy sex.

Very often it is possible in therapy with such men to find out why it is that they become attached to the object, although the fetish may be entirely harmless.

WHEN DOES A FETISH START?
A particular fetish almost always dates back to very early in life or to around the time when a child first started to masturbate. There is little doubt that

fetishism is to a great extent a learned phenomenon and that as a boy starts to incorporate ideas and images of women as meaningful sex objects, he can be influenced in his ideas as he learns to masturbate.

So it is that a boy might experience his first masturbatory experiences to the accompaniment of a certain picture, fantasy object or woman. His mind then becomes 'locked' into this image which remains a very powerful stimulus for him whenever he wants to become turned on quickly.

RESTRICTIONS
The trouble with this, and indeed with all fetishes, is that they are somewhat restricting. It is rather like being able to obtain one's pleasure from a tiny number of very rare foods. This would mean that one could only really enjoy a meal at a few restaurants in the whole country and would have to seek them out. So it is with fetishes. They restrict the individual's choice both of activities and sex partners. This may or may not prove to be a problem, depending on the nature of the fetish. Obviously, some fetishes are a great deal easier to accommodate than others.

TYPES OF FETISH

There are two main types of fetish. In the first, the man is 'into' inanimate objects such as leather, rubber, underwear, shoes and so on. In the other, he is obsessed with a part of a woman's body only, for example her bottom – or indeed bottoms in general.

This latter is less common and varies greatly in different parts of the world. For example, in most parts of the world, a woman's breasts are not considered to be sex objects, they are organs for feeding babies. In many such cultures, the buttocks are thought to be much more sexy. In the West, though, many men are heavily 'into breasts' yet we do not call them fetishists, although men in other cultures might do so.

A MALE PRESERVE

Perhaps the most interesting thing about fetishes is that they are, unlike almost anything else in human sexuality, an almost entirely male interest. Just why this should be is not known but it is fascinating to find that as women are becoming more free in their sexuality they too are starting to have fetishes.

A NARROW VIEW

Adolescent boys are more open to the use of erotic and soft pornography, both of which enable them to centre their fantasies and conscious thoughts on women, parts of women, and fetishistic objects as they learn to masturbate. Girls very rarely do this because their interest tends to be more personality centred – on

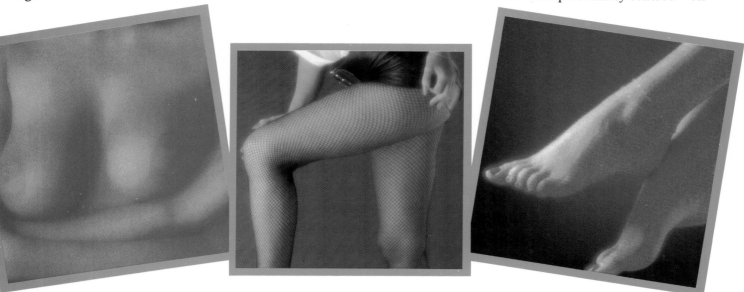

MAGICAL POWERS

The original use of the word fetish was in the context of an object that was thought to have magical powers. This was certainly so in many African cultures. It was not until late in the nineteenth century that the meaning of the word was changed to incorporate a sexual meaning. Now it is almost always used to mean a pursuit of some kind to which an individual is devoted or compulsively drawn. It still has a magical overtone to it and many men say that they feel inexplicably drawn, as if in some mystical way, to their fetishistic object.

But more common than this is the interest in, and sexual need for, things which only have oblique connections with women. Anything can become a fetishistic object, but the most common of these are leather, rubber, fur, silk, underwear, women's shoes, boots and gloves. Some men like to dress up in clothes that are inappropiate for them. This can take the form of transvestism or cross-dressing (dressing up in women's clothes) or even dressing in uniforms or children's clothes. There is almost always a strong psychosexual reason for these needs.

the man in whom they are interested – rather than on sexual things or parts of men as 'objects'. Just how much of this is biological and how much purely cultural is difficult to know. Whatever the explanation, it will be a very long time before women are as affected by fetishes as are men. This could be said to be a good thing because, while it may be pleasant to be able to find sexual pleasure from many sources, some of which might even be inanimate, if these involve a member of the opposite sex it can be restricting because one has to find someone with similar interests or a partner who will tolerate them.

FETISHISM AND MORALITY

Many a moralist is against all forms of fetishism involving inanimate objects because, they argue, sex is an interpersonal pastime and that to have a 'sexual relationship' with a shoe or something similar is somehow degrading to both the individual and to women in general.

But whatever people's views about fetishes, and many women find the whole subject quite difficult because they are, by and large, turned on by men as people and not as objects, they are here to stay and will continue to form at least a part of the sexual life of a great many men. If they can be accommodated within a man-woman relationship (whether he involves her directly or not in its pursuit), then all is well.

UNDERWEAR

Fetishes and fantasies about underwear and actually finding underwear highly arousing in real life are not uncommon. It is not known for sure why this should be but there are several possible explanations.

First, it could be simply that underwear covers up the really interesting sexual parts of a woman's body. Many a woman says that she feels more sexy and sexually arousing to the opposite sex when dressed only in underwear than when naked. It has much to do with the promise of things to come and to the leaving of the best until last. It also focuses attention on the covered parts in a way that total nakedness does not.

Women's underwear is also often pretty to look at and is designed to be visually attractive to both sexes whether the man who is looking at it is an underwear fetishist or not.

BACK TO CHILDHOOD
But perhaps the most interesting explanation of the fascination that so many men have for partly-clad women goes back to childhood. Around the age of three or so, it becomes clear to many mothers that their little boys are becoming more than casually interested in their mother's body. This is a time when most of us go through a stage when we are interested in our opposite-sex parent and can even become quite jealous of the same-sex parent. Some little girls are 'heavily into daddy' at this age and wish their mother would go away – some even wish her dead.

THE INFLUENCE OF THE MOTHER
Boys, too, have such feelings towards their mothers and feel a sense of rivalry towards their fathers. The mother who would, and probably did, previously go around the house naked is now encouraged by both her husband and her own self-consciousness to put at least some clothes on. It is suggested by some psychoanalysts who have examined the matter that little boys at this stage of their psychosexual development now come to find the sight of their mothers in their underwear highly attractive and that this image lasts with them for the rest of their lives.

Just how much of such a man's later fixation on underwear has to do with his unconscious yearnings for his mother is open to debate but it is not nearly as fanciful as it might at first appear.

Some mothers, for reasons which at the time seem justifiable to them, are over-close to their young boys. This can occur if the husband is away on business, in prison, or in hospital for a long period. The mother,

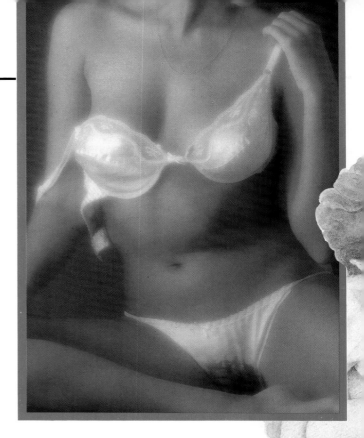

For the man with a breast fetish, caressing them can be more exciting if the woman remains partially clothed, thus exaggerating her shape – and perhaps size

A fetish for shoes, boots or any item of clothing can be simply incorporated into a couple's repertoire if the woman wears the specific garment during lovemaking. For her, remaining partially clothed can be almost as stimulating as are his sensations when they make love

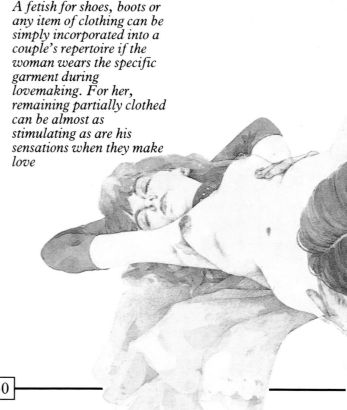

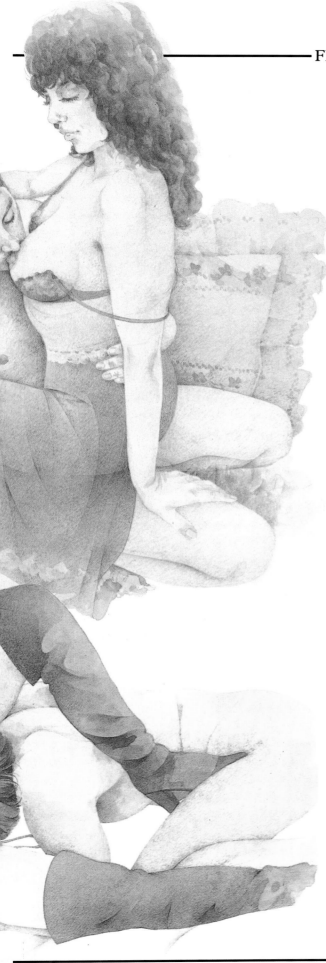

quite unconsciously in the vast majority of cases, takes the child over as if he were a replacement for her lost man and makes him into 'her little man'. If this persists, he is too closely bound to her and her needs – the relationship after all is not forged because of his needs but because of her own.

Such a boy is then in trouble later as his peers become independent of their mothers while he remains firmly tied to her. Strangely enough, exactly the same thing can occur if the woman rejects her boy – he then clings to her, but for the opposite reasons.

THE UNCONSCIOUS MIND

As with all fetishes, women in general, or the woman in the man's life, are at least to some extent represented by the objects involved. This helps to explain why it is that so many men find underwear so sexy both in fact and fantasy. Some men, however unconsciously, are clinging on to memories, long since banished from consciousness, of other women they have known in real life, or those from pages of women's magazines or in advertisements. Perhaps some time long ago, these memories were locked into their sexual unconscious to reside there ready to be activated by a woman in underwear whether she is his real partner, or simply a fantasy.

RIGHTS AND WRONGS

In a sense, then, the underwear is being made love to and not the woman.

But before women throw up their hands in horror and say how disgusting this is, it is worth bearing in mind that research shows that the majority of women when making love fantasize about something, often nothing at all to do with their partner. It cannot be 'right' for women to do this and 'wrong' for men to fantasize about fetishistic objects . . . at least few honest people would accept such hypocrisy. To some extent, we all make use of fantasy material to enhance our lovemaking and the loving couple finds ways of enriching their sex lives and that of their partner the best way they can.

A woman who knows that her partner has such a fetish can easily help him to indulge it. She can send off for lingerie catalogues that they both then discuss. He will undoubtedly use the pictures as aids to masturbation and they could even do this together. She can dress in underwear that he particularly likes or she can model for him to take photos of her as if she were going to appear in one of the catalogues.

AN ACCEPTABLE WAY

Indeed, such a woman is lucky because her man's fetish is easily catered for in a socially acceptable way. Even having to make love with her in her underwear is no great problem for the average woman. Things are not so easy, though, for the partner of the man who has another kind of fantasy. Fetishes involving rubber are complex to explain but tend to be more widespread than would be first thought.

A DISTINCTIVE SMELL

The first explanation, and one that is rarely advanced, is that there could be something in rubber that is attractive to men's senses. Perhaps some men are aroused by one of the many chemicals that go into the making of rubber. We know so little about smells and their effect on the body, but it is at least possible that there are chemicals that are given off in imperceptibly tiny amounts which then affect certain men sexually. Rubber, after all, has a very distinctive smell.

EARLY IN INFANCY

Chemical explanations aside, there are very plausible psychological mechanisims that could be at play.

Early in life, some men who have such a fetish will have come across rubber in the setting of their babyhood. They will have had a rubber sheet or rubber pants over their nappies, and it is not unreasonable to suggest that these objects take on a meaning that is linked to their mother and her caring and loving behaviour.

It is also possible that the very distinctive feel and smell of the rubber then becomes bound to the emotional and psychological images of the mother and what she stands for. It might even symbolize the comfort of the cot the little boy once lay in. Most children grow out of this association, at least consciously, but some go on to stay with the smell and feel of the rubber and it becomes built into their sexual and sensual personality.

Many a child of either sex clings on to a blanket or toy as a reminder of its mother when she is not there. Such things are called 'transitional objects' by psychologists. They come to represent the mother who is out of sight, perhaps downstairs at night, or when she is out at work or away in hospital. The child comforts itself with the blanket or whatever it is and becomes extremely distressed if anyone threatens to remove it.

If such a transitional object is made of rubber it is not hard to see that it could have a lasting significance to the child.

A SOCIAL STIGMA

The problem with rubber fetishes, and indeed with many fetishes, is that they can be somewhat difficult to indulge. Few grown men, in fact, enjoy a rubber sheet or toy such as they had when they were little, and finding alternatives that are associated with women can be difficult, especially for the bashful. Specialist mail-order catalogues are widely available but many men feel ashamed and so do not send off for them.

The trouble arises if they need or want their partner to indulge in the fantasy fetish with them. A few women are game to do so, but many are not and cannot understand why it is that their man cannot manage 'straight' sex with them.

Of course, he usually can. Most men with a fetish are not in a position of being unable to enjoy sex without the fetishistic object or part of woman's anatomy – they simply do not find nearly so much

A fetish for underwear can be easily catered for by the loving couple. Loose-fitting or crotchless panties not only look and feel sexy – they allow easy access to, and penetration of, the vagina

pleasure out of normal sex. Some, of course, have no partner either because they are unmarried or because their partner is unavailable to them. Such men usually retreat to their particular fetish as their only form of enhancer during masturbation.

FINDING A SOLUTION

Simply dressing up in rubber gear of some kind may be no great hardship from time to time for a woman wanting to please, but quite a few rubber fetishists also enjoy other things such as sado-masochistic pursuits or 'water games'. These are much less attractive to most women, so the man who wants his partner to help him indulge his rubber fetish might have to keep such other interests strictly limited to his fantasy life.

The devoted fetishist, however, will not be satisfied and will seek out other women, perhaps a prostitute, to answer these more unusual needs.

GROUP SEX FANTASIES

Who fantasizes about group sex? What is its attraction? And is there any way such fantasies can be simply incorporated into a couple's lovemaking?

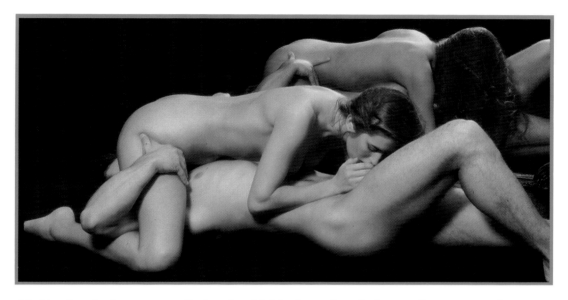

Making love in the presence of others is a highly charged erotic fantasy for many couples

To many people, the notion of a sexual encounter that involves more than just their partner is highly exciting. Indeed, some form of group sexual activity is a common fantasy in both sexes. In the 'swinging '60s', much was said about group sex and many people experimented with it. But over the following decade it fell out of fashion, because most of those who tried it found that it was disappointing and held little of value for them except as a novelty.

THE SANDSTONE EXPERIMENT
Perhaps the most sophisticated and well-documented example of group sex was at a private home called Sandstone in California. This large estate had a beautiful house that the owners made available to all couples who wanted to go there on a club-like basis to make love in the presence of others.

Nudity was the norm at most times and in the evenings couples gathered together in one of two enormous rooms where they would talk, cuddle and make love if they wanted. For most of those going there, it was their first experience of open sexuality, certainly with their full-time partners.

CHANGING PARTNERS
Couples changed partners if they wanted to and the any-thing-goes atmosphere was conducive to losing inhibitions on a grand scale. Homosexual contacts between men were very rare but, perhaps surprisingly, they were common between women. Sex-play tended to be conventional and most people made love in fairly conventional ways too. Some men brought their very reluctant partners only to find that the women ended up enjoying it considerably more than the men did.

A NEW EXPERIENCE
Few people can predict how they will respond to a group sex encounter, but it is a favourite fantasy subject for many of us. When asked, most men on their first visit to Sandstone were found to be highly stimulated by the idea of group sex but were very concerned that they would not perform adequately. Women were worried that the experience might be dangerous or distasteful, or that they would find themselves having to have sex with men they did not fancy. Jointly, couples were worried about how they would cope with feeling of jealousy.

The vast majority of these fears proved to be unfounded and the experience caused no problems at all for most of the couples involved.

NOT TYPICAL

Yet the members of Sandstone were far from typical Americans. They were intelligent, educated, liberal and open to new experiences – and they were volunteers. And it is quite possible that there were more long-term problems than were recorded at the time. It would be interesting to follow up such a group twenty years on and see what they think now.

JEALOUSY

Most couples who have experience of group sex find that jealousy plays a negative role in the proceedings. This is especially true for men who, seeing their usual partner greatly enjoying herself in the arms of another man, become jealous because he does not realize that she is more turned on than usual because of the novelty of the situation. He invariably thinks it is because the other man is a better lover and this can lead to trouble.

This type of misunderstanding arises because we are all brought up to be somewhat over-private when it comes to our bodies and our sexuality. Some sex therapists believe that a certain amount of sexual openness, perhaps with true friends with whom a couple feels at ease, would help at least some people become less inhibited, thus relaxing them.

LEARNING THROUGH WATCHING

Sex has a large learned component to it for all humans. Many women, seeing another becoming orgasmic, or even truly enjoying sex, can be greatly aroused and become more willing to try more adventurous pursuits themselves. They may believe that they are the only ones with earthy needs and, as a result, feel guilty for wanting to express them.

A much simpler way of achieving the same result can be found by watching erotic films – many such films contain highly explicit scenes involving group sex. This is probably safer because it does not actually involve revealing one's personal sexuality to other people and allows one to be a voyeur.

Certainly, group sex demolishes myths about age and good looks. Once it becomes apparent that the old and ugly can have beautiful sex, it is difficult to cling on to such stereotypes for long.

THE DANGERS

At Sandstone, most couples said that they found watching their partner being made love to by someone else highly stimulating and not at all threatening. This is, however, rather different from most situations involving group sex where only one other couple is present. This situation – usually called swinging – is potentially much more dangerous because, unlike the Sandstone experiment, the situation is open to long-term relationships developing with all the attendant

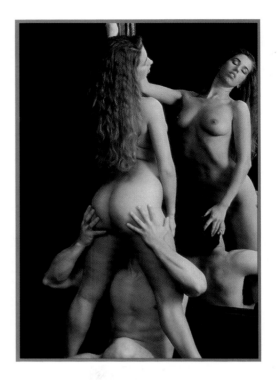

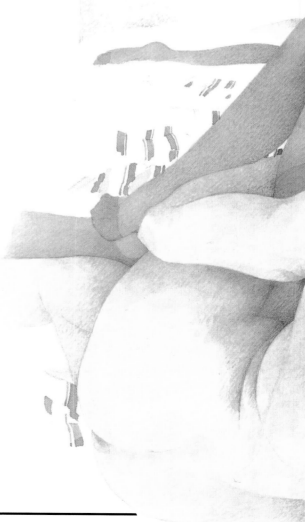

problems. In any form of group sex, the couple who are 'ticking over' in their relationship often find apparent sexual fulfilment within the group and this can kill off the relationship.

A PRACTICAL SOLUTION

It seems, therefore, that the disadvantages to group sex outweigh the advantages. A few people will always want to try it, if only for the novelty of the situation, but it is unlikely to become a way of life for any but the tiniest of minorities. It is probably safest, therefore, to keep group sex to the realms of fantasy, which is exactly what most people do.

TWO WOMEN

Many men find the idea of two women making love attractive – indeed it is a classical soft-porn image in

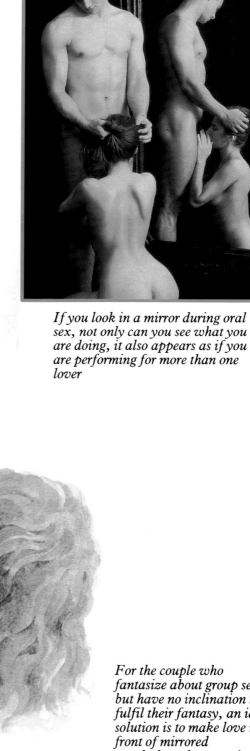

If you look in a mirror during oral sex, not only can you see what you are doing, it also appears as if you are performing for more than one lover

For the couple who fantasize about group sex but have no inclination to fulfil their fantasy, an ideal solution is to make love in front of mirrored wardrobes, thus creating the illusion of another couple being there too

Rear-entry positions were once thought to be immoral – for the man who fantasizes about anal sex, however, or who is particularly turned on by the sight of his partner's buttocks, they can be favourite positions for lovemaking

(right) A loving couple can create their own personal sex orgy if they are prepared to use their imagination to the full – making love in a rear-entry position and watching a blue movie at the same time is one practice that couples may find highly arousing

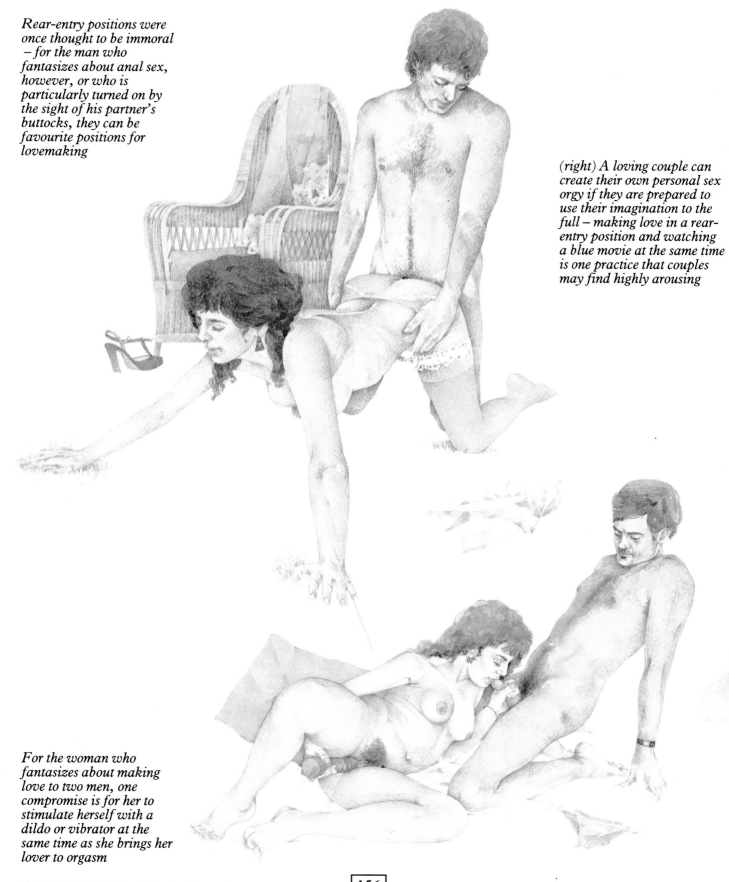

For the woman who fantasizes about making love to two men, one compromise is for her to stimulate herself with a dildo or vibrator at the same time as she brings her lover to orgasm

magazines and films. It is as if another woman will be able to teach a man how better to excite his woman, but the attraction goes beyond this for many men. Women are exciting to look at naked on their own but two silky soft, sensuous bodies playing and loving is a very powerful turn-on to most men.

This is often totally impossible to arrange in real life but can just about be achieved if there are two

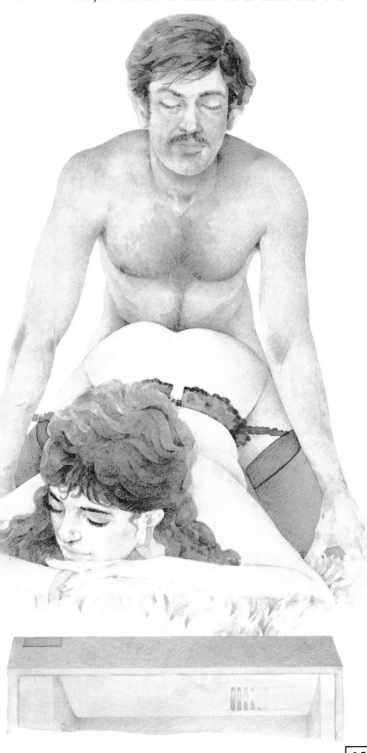

couples involved and the girls caress each other. This could well be a conscious, if not unconscious, reason behind some men's thrills at foursomes.

SHARING ONE'S PARTNER
Given that sex is so private and that other people's sexual lives are thus all the more fascinating, it is hardly surprising that simply watching another couple making love, even if it does not involve swapping partners, would be likely to be both arousing and interesting. There are few events and pastimes in life that we cannot and do not share with our friends and acquaintances, but sex remains intensely personal and private.

This is really what many pornographic films and videos cater for. There is always the hope that one's own behaviour will be confirmed as normal and that one might pick up a tip or two to improve one's own technique, performance or enjoyment. In fact, it is rather like watching a professional golf tournament if you are an amateur enthusiast.

DISSATISFACTION
The dangers are many in foursomes because in such a small group there is a real possibility that serious interpersonal bonds could form and that these could threaten the original love bonds of the couples.

It is easy too, given that the situation is novel and highly arousing, that any one of the four could think that this kind of sex was better than just with his or her partner. This can lead to long-term dissatisfaction and marital breakups. Most people have more inhibitions than they thought and soon find the total 'freedom' of group sex somewhat alarming or destructive.

COMPARING OURSELVES WITH OTHERS
We all tend to compare ourselves with others and many women are very sensitive to their bodies being unattractive to themselves or their men. One study, for example, found that more than 70 per cent of women were dissatisfied with their breasts. Imagine then how a women who thought this way could adversely compare herself if her partner were seen to be greatly turned on by a woman whom she considered to have better breasts than her own. Much the same argument goes for penis size in men.

BETTER IN FANTASY
In general, group sex appeals more to men than to women, although fantasies of having sex with multiple partners (a 'gang bang') is much more common in women than men. Yet some men are impotent in their first encounter with group sex and this can continue into their one-to-one relationships later.

Group sex and orgies are probably better kept to the world of fantasy than dragged into real life. Most happily-bonded and well-adjusted couples do not need such diversions and, if they do, can often find some imaginative, and safe, way of incorporating them into their sex lives together.

WHEN THINGS GO WRONG

When problems arise in a loving relationship, the couple's store of sexual goodwill can do much to solve any difficulties

---

From time to time, things go wrong in even the most loving couple's sex life. For the man, it can result in premature ejaculation or temporary impotence, while a woman may stop having orgasms altogether. Lovers who have been together for some time and who enjoy inventive and satisfactory sex together are more capable of sorting most of these problems out when they arise.

HOW CAN THINGS GO WRONG?

The vast majority of sexual problems take place in the mind of one or both partners. Humans are complicated

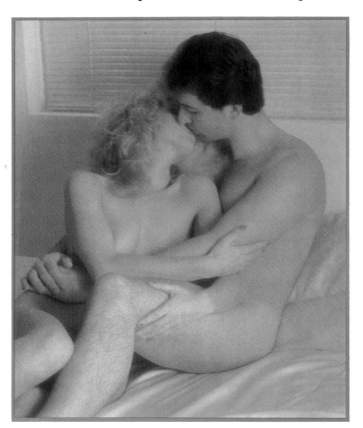

beings and nowhere is this more clearly demonstrated than in the field of sexual relationships. Sex can be fantastic one day and the next the magic seems to have gone. If that magic fails to re-appear during the next session of lovemaking, and then the next, the feeling of failure slots in the mind. The subconscious efficiently files it away and, naturally, the couple starts to worry. That worry begins to nag away and before the couple know it they have a problem of impotence or frigidity on their hands and this can put a strain on their relationship.

MALE WORRIES

The man is in a rather worse position that his partner when things start to go wrong. If a woman suddenly stops experiencing orgasm, it does not prevent her from having sex. But if a man fails to achieve an erection or he comes too soon, the result is there for all to see. Certainly he can make his partner come by using his hands or his mouth but, for him, the experience will not end in orgasm. If he does not understand his problem, the chances are that he will continue to worry even as he concentrates on his partner's needs.

And whether we like it ot not, many men are concerned about 'performance' in bed. No amount of counselling can take away from such a man's mind that somehow he is the doer, sexually. The visibility of his situation probably only makes the matter worse. And if he comes too soon, he cannot fake orgasm as a woman is able to.

THE PERFORMANCE MYTH

The modern male lover has a great deal to live up to. Fifty years ago and more, male performance in bed, or lack of it, was not recognized – or, if it was, it was not discussed.

Whatever the real-life sexuality during the Victorian

For whatever reasons, when things go wrong, a loving touch and an appreciation of each other's sensuality will go a long way towards putting things right

---

era, it is almost certainly true to say that the sex act was over and done with much more quickly than it is today. Because the female body was always covered, men were inevitably highly aroused when it was exposed – even part of it. One popular Victorian novel describes its hero being overcome at the sight of a woman's dimpled elbow.

More importantly, sexual repression meant that men had no need for sexual technique, and a woman's satisfaction was considered irrelevant to the sex act – if indeed it was considered in any way at all.

Nowadays, the reverse is true. Women are, quite rightly, concerned with their own sexual satisfaction and the man is there to ensure that this happens. In many relationships, the man puts his own satisfaction below that of his partner. And the modern male stereotypes in literature and the media never fail to deliver the goods – their penises are giant sized and permanently erect, they embark on marathon love-making sessions where the woman's orgasms just keep on coming, and their ejaculations are perfectly timed with incredible power. In reality, no man can live up to the myth.

FEMALE MYTHS
In a different way from men, the modern woman also has a great deal to live up to. Just as men have to live up to the performances of their media prototypes, women are supposed to have a voracious appetite when it comes to sex. They are always ready and

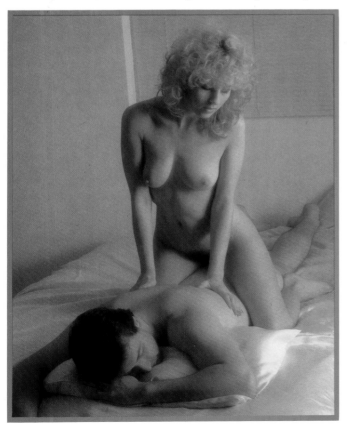

willing, their orgasms are frequent – often they are multi-orgasmic. They love oral sex and they willingly take the lead. Add to that the well-endowed bodies that stare out from the magazines – together with the endless streams of prose in agony columns and fiction promoting sexual promiscuity on one hand and constant fidelity on the other, and it is hardly surprising that the modern woman is in a sexual dilemma. But, unlike men, she really has no way of knowing exactly what is expected of her.

THE MODERN COUPLE
The advanced couple recognizes the myths and has probably worked out where they stand, but no one is immune from sexual exploitation. The point is we all want to be good in bed, but this is not something that happens overnight, as if by magic.

Good sex has to be learned and practised – preferably regularly and with the same loving partner. Most of us recognize that good sex rarely happens the first time that a couple sleep together – the best sex comes through familiarity with each other.

A problem of premature ejaculation can be concealed once or twice but cannot be kept permanently from the discerning eyes of a long-term partner. Equally, a woman's orgasm can be faked to please on a one-night stand, but under the loving gaze of her regular lover it will soon become clear that there is something wrong.

WHAT CAN A COUPLE DO?
A person who is experiencing short-term sexual problems can be helped by the understanding of his or her partner. As with any other problem, the solving can be done together. If the man is experiencing difficulties, the woman can use her body, hands and mouth and, more importantly, her head to help him. And in the same way, the man can use patience and understanding to help his partner through any difficulties that she may have.

In the vast majority of cases, a loving partner is the best sex therapist. And because sex is fun, the solving of the problem can then become a memorable and affectionate way of increasing the scope of a couple's sex lives together. And, as always, the advanced lover puts love and consideration of the other's needs before sexual technique.

HER FOR HIM

Although there can be any number of reasons why a man may experience sexual difficulties, it generally shows itself in one of two ways. Either he comes too soon, or he takes too long, sometimes not managing to come at all. The answer to either problem is not be found solely in the sexual technique of his partner, although it is going to help. More important will be her willingness to help him overcome the problem – to turn it into a shared challenge.

First of all, she will need to be prepared to talk – and then to listen. Perhaps the man needs to be reassured, flattered or spoilt. Perhaps he is worried, stressed or has a problem at work. Whatever the reason, he needs to be encouraged to communicate about it. The advanced couple will recognize this and will make communication, romance and so on part of foreplay which in turn will serve to lessen the problem before taking the next physical step.

TAKE THE PRESSURE OFF

In a good majority of cases where the man's performance lets him and his partner down, the difficulties he is experiencing are often a direct result of the pressure he feels to 'perform' sexually. It is up to the woman to help him to reduce that pressure and, preferably, make it disappear altogether.

The best way of doing this is to tell your partner that this is what you want to do. Tell him that he does not need to worry about your pleasure for the time being. Tell him that it is not unmasculine to lie there and enjoy himself once in a while. Love should transcend those barriers anyway.

WHEN HE COMES TOO SOON

Most men suffer from premature ejaculation at some time in their lives. Rather than regarding it as a problem, the woman can take responsibility to treat it in a number of ways. She can give him an orgasm before they make love, she can use the squeeze technique, or she can use a form of controlled intercourse called stop-start. Preferably, she can try a mixture of all three. But whichever method she uses, the golden rule is to make what is happening fun.

GIVE HIM AN EARLY ORGASM

Lie your partner back and use your hands to give him an early orgasm – not with your mouth, which may be too arousing for him. The aim of this early orgasm, paradoxically, is to make it as low-key as possible. Use both hands to slowly rub his penis. As his orgasm approaches, resist the temptation to rub faster and harder. Just keep the same slow rhythm going until he ejaculates. Then use your mouth to re-arouse him to make love – his next orgasm should take much longer.

THE SQUEEZE GAME

The advanced couple will probably be familiar with the squeeze technique which unfortunately often smacks of problems and sexual disaster. But for the man who comes too soon it does work – more importantly, it can be fun.

To begin with, settle back into a comfortable position and start to masturbate him, slowly at first, and bring him to the brink of orgasm. Agree a signal

Consideration for each other's needs will help any couple through sexual problems. Devote yourself to those particular aspects of lovemaking your partner finds most arousing

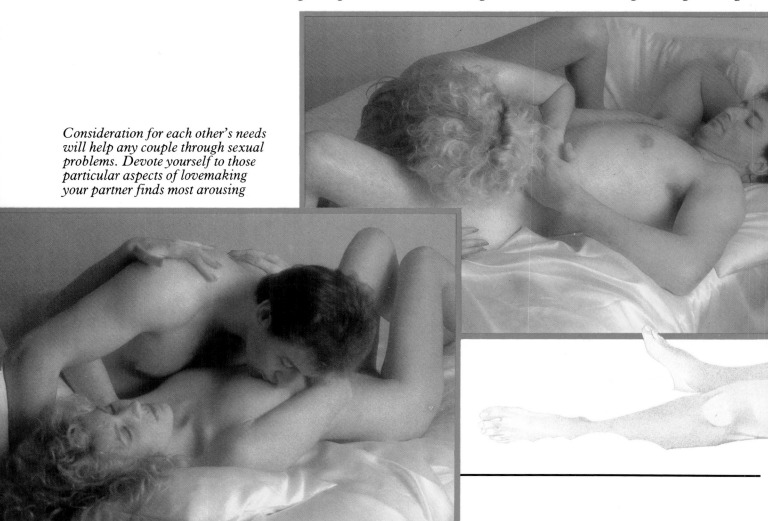

that his orgasm is approaching – or quite simply, get him to tell you when it is coming. Stop stimulating him and squeeze the tip of his penis firmly with your thumb over the little ridge on its underside and two other fingers on the opposite side of its rim. Squeeze hard for about 15 to 20 seconds and he should immediately lose his erection.

TAKE TIME
Now use your mouth on his penis as skilfully as possible and bring him back to the brink of orgasm – it should take slightly longer, this time. Again, just before the point of no return, take his penis out of your mouth and squeeze it hard. If he has managed to increase the length of time before his climax approaches use one of the woman-on-top positions and bring him to orgasm.

The secret now is to continue the programme. Use your mouth as skilfully as you know how to revive him and, when his erection is firm, take a woman-on-top position and make love to him again. The golden rule is to ensure that he does not feel that he needs to 'perform'. And if he wants you to have an orgasm yourself, encourage him to use his hands or mouth – or a vibrator – whichever you both prefer.

STOP-START
The key to controlling the time of the man's orgasm during actual intercourse is for the woman to take up a position where she is totally in control, and for this a woman-on-top position is ideal as the man's thrusting can be kept to a minimum.

It is obviously best to use a position where you are facing him rather than facing away so that you can gauge his reactions. Lie him back on the bed and straddle him, support yourself on your hands beside him and take his penis into your vagina, but only a little way. Now keep it still. Talk to him and try to discourage him from thinking about what you are doing which he will probably find too arousing – get him to try and concentrate on anything else. And control any temptation to move your lower body. Now, take him in a little deeper and start to move your buttocks slowly. If he feels he is about to come, withdraw from him immediately until the sensation passes before continuing the process.

A bonus of this technique for many women is that they may find it highly arousing themselves, although this is a double-edged sword in that the more aroused you become, the more will he. A way round this is to continue so that he has his orgasm and then to use your hands or mouth on him and start doing the same thing all over again.

Getting this right could take anything up to two months, but the loving couple should recognize that this is an effective – and fruitful – way of investing their sexual time together. The woman can also content herself with the knowledge that, soon, her lover will be all that she wants in bed.

FAILURE TO COME
For the man who starts to experience difficulties in having an orgasm, the first thing to do is to stop

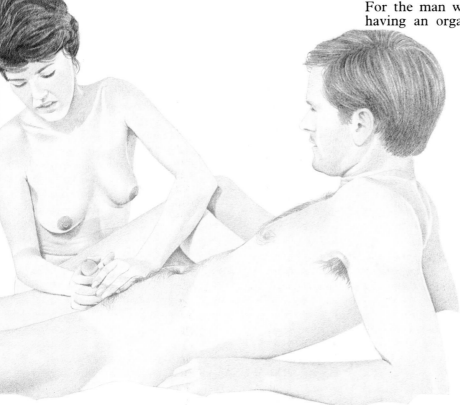

When premature ejaculation is the problem, bringing your partner to orgasm before attempting intercourse is one solution – but keep his initial orgasm low-key

having conventional intercourse. This is a slightly more tricky problem for the woman to solve than if the man is coming too soon, but again it can be made fun – and not just for her partner.

Initially, you will need to place greater emphasis on his arousal – kiss more, cuddle more and increase your general closeness together. Your partner will almost certainly be worried and you need to take the pressure off him.

When you go to bed together, practice creative foreplay but do not, in these early stages, touch his genitals. Use erotic massage and get him to do the same to you. Encourage him to become excited again by your body, although do not be tempted to move ahead too quickly.

MUTUAL MASTURBATION

Encourage him to watch you masturbate so that he becomes aroused – allow him to bring you to orgasm like this if he want to. Teach him what you like best. Encourage him to masturbate himself and note what gives him pleasure; get him to tell you what he particularly enjoys. Then see if you can reproduce the sensations he has given himself. If he wants to, let him concentrate on giving you pleasure which should help to take his mind off his own sensations.

USE ORAL SEX

The loving couple will have made oral sex part of their loveplay together and will know that it is always an effective way of bringing a man to orgasm, especially if he is taking too long during conventional intercourse. Encourage him not to worry and just to enjoy the sensations of your mouth, tongue and lips as you use them on his penis to slowly bring him to his climax. To arouse him still further, use a 69 position where you get on top of him. The sight of your vulva and the sensations that he experiences as he uses his mouth on you should dramatically increase the level of his arousal. Use your hands elsewhere on his body as well, perhaps stroking his perineum or his buttocks.

IN INTERCOURSE

Provided that your partner is managing to maintain an erection, now is the time to get him to make love to you. Explain to him that it is not vital for your own pleasure that he comes – the Chinese practised non-ejaculatory intercourse for centuries as a means of satisfying their partners, so there is no reason why he should not do the same. Allow him to take a position where he is in control and where the quality of his erection is not too important – his confidence has to be paramount at this point. Lie down on the bed while he is in a kneeling position, get him to put his hands under your buttocks and lift you up to him – wrap your legs around his waist. This will enable him to move from side to side to stimulate his penis and avoid any danger of his penis slipping out.

If he fails to come, lovingly use your mouth on his penis to bring him to orgasm.

HIM FOR HER

Suddenly, after a rich and varied sex life with her partner, a woman may find that she has difficulty in coming. There can be a host of reasons why this should be so and most can be solved with the help of a loving partner. The reason behind any such problem, however, is often more difficult to find than if a man experiences difficulties because, although a woman's

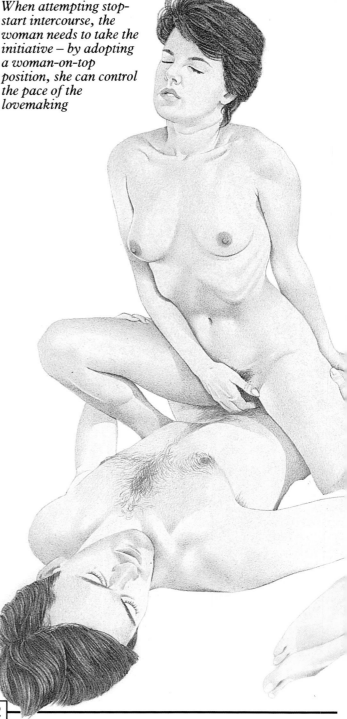

When attempting stop-start intercourse, the woman needs to take the initiative – by adopting a woman-on-top position, she can control the pace of the lovemaking

potential may be higher than a man's, she is also vulnerable to a wider range of potential sexual difficulties. Yet, more often than not, the answer is only too simple – the form of contraception she is using, the recent birth of a baby, pre-menstrual tension and so on. But whatever the reason, she is going to need help and consideration from her partner to restore her sexuality.

SEDUCE HER

Even the most loving relationships can become sexually stale after a while, and this is the time for the man to take the opportunity of turning the clock back and treating his partner as he did in the early days of their courtship.

To many women, lovemaking is less about sex and more about the emotional and mental approach to it. If that is right, then the rest should follow. The tried and tested means of seduction invariably work, especially if they appear in a slightly new context. So take your partner out to dinner, get her to dress so that she feels good, perhaps give her a small present and concentrate on making the whole evening memorable.

USE FOREPLAY

Linger on foreplay as long as you can and be inventive. Use your hands and mouth, try a vibrator or dildo or whatever you know she really likes. Kiss her, talk to her and concentrate on making her feel sexy.

Make taking off her clothes as sensual as you can, bath or shower her and then, as erotically as you can, give her a massage. When you make love to her, choose a position that you know she likes, but

concentrate on making the lovemaking slow and sensual – do not hurry anything. It is not one individual component, but all of them coming together in the right way, that makes lovemaking memorable for her. Forget your own needs – they should be satisfied by the increased level of your arousal anyway.

CHOOSE A POSITION

Most positions have something special going for them but the side-entry position is one of the best positions for relaxing intercourse. Use your penis and your hands to kiss and cuddle her and caress her clitoris. Tell her that you want to give her pleasure.

If the tempo needs increasing, then you can try to change the mood entirely and let her set the pace. Lie back and get her to sit astride you, but facing away, and get her to use her body to give herself pleasure. Encourage her to fantasize and use her hands on herself to bring herself to orgasm.

USE AFTERPLAY

To set the scene for the next time you make love, use creative afterplay. After lovemaking, kiss and caress her. Tell her how much you love and want her. Kiss her breasts and, if she becomes aroused, start all over again. Make it obvious that it is her pleasure you are seeking and that yours is found in providing that pleasure for her.

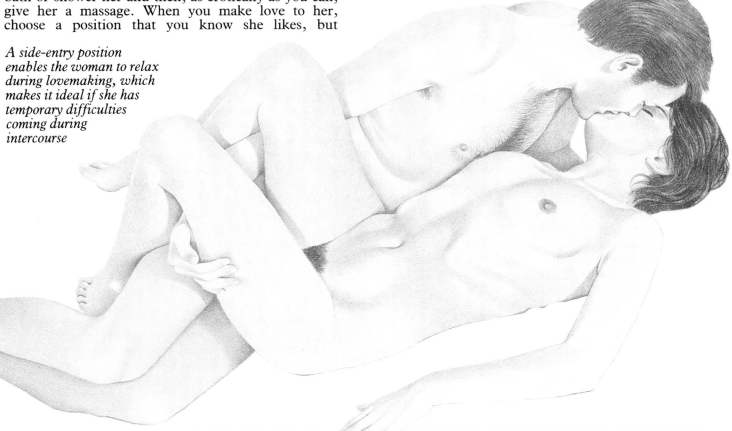

A side-entry position enables the woman to relax during lovemaking, which makes it ideal if she has temporary difficulties coming during intercourse

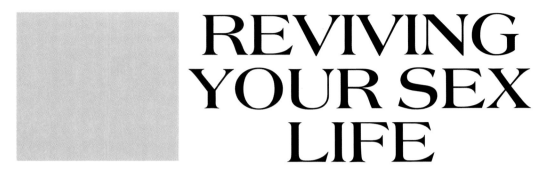

REVIVING YOUR SEX LIFE

Sexual boredom can set in to even the best of loving relationships,
but excitement can be restored with a little imagination and effort

There are few relationships which are so perfect that they do not undergo a period when one or both partners feel that their sex life is becoming just a little stale. Yet, provided that the couple still love each other, there are plenty of things they can do to restore their love life – and even improve it. It is all a question of approach.

WHY DOES GOOD SEX DETERIORATE?

It is an extraordinary relationship that can maintain the sexual enthusiasm of the very early days together. Most men and women are just not built to withstand the trauma and excitement of that phase on a permanent basis. Tiredness, a young family, pressures of work – both in and out of the home – can all seem to conspire to make satisfying sex certainly less regular and often something to be got over with as quickly as possible.

What makes the cause of declining sex more difficult to identify for the couple concerned is that the process does not happen overnight. The changes are almost imperceptible because they happen so slowly, and a couple that has been making love almost every night at the start of a relationship may gradually find they do it only once or twice a week.

This in itself may not matter if the couple are happy with such a state of affairs – provided the quality of the lovemaking remains satisfactory this may well suit both of them. The problems start to arise when one partner starts to feel sexually discontented.

SECURITY

For a couple who have been together for a few years, there are many compensations in their lives. They are familiar with each other's emotional and sexual needs, they know exactly how to turn each other on and there is a feeling of 'safeness' and security in the relationship – qualities that are important to both sexes.

Yet perhaps this very security conspires to affect a couple's sex life. For many people it is often the illicitness of sex rather than the sex itself, that makes it so attractive. There is, perhaps, a need for risk in all of us.

WHAT CAN A COUPLE DO?

If a couple sit down and start to examine what is going wrong with their sex life they may well come to realize that the actual sex itself is still satisfactory. What is almost certainly missing is the build-up and the foreplay that would have been such a feature of their early sexual life together.

Yet the word foreplay covers a multitude of presexual gambits. It can start in the morning with sex taking place in the evening, it can be a word spoken, a gift, a kiss or caress. The beginnings of arousal – particularly for women – take place when the man announces his intentions. Physical closeness through the day, a small bunch of flowers – almost anything can be used to arouse one's partner.

THE EARLY DAYS

A couple who complain of a flagging sex life are best advised to look back to the physical closeness of their early days together. It is all too easy to neglect touching, kissing and attentiveness, yet it is these things that can make or break lovemaking and determine its ultimate quality.

SET ASIDE SOME TIME

Research has shown that one of the greatest criticisms women have of their partners, sexually, is that they do not take enough time. Behind this complaint is probably not so much a criticism of their partner's actual sexual technique when they are making love; the complaint reflects more the lack of attention to courtship details that most men, early on in a relationship, are all too ready to give.

Similarly, the most common male complaint is that their partner is not as sexually exciting as she was in the early days of their relationship.

If a relationship is doomed anyway, then these complaints can become impenetrable barriers to a couple's future sexual happiness. But for most of us, the answer lies – as it does in so many other areas of human relationship – in some sort of compromise and fully understanding the needs of our partner.

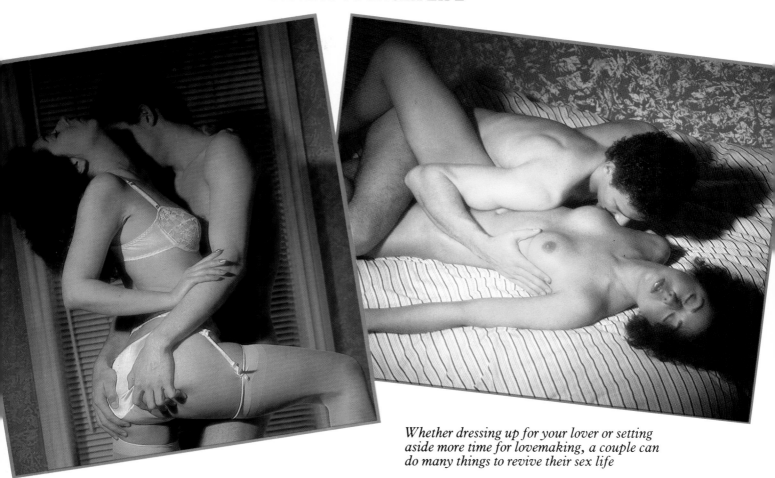

Whether dressing up for your lover or setting aside more time for lovemaking, a couple can do many things to revive their sex life

HOW TO COMPROMISE

For the man, a return to courtship behaviour is an attitude of mind – once he decides what he will do, the rest is straightforward. After all, it will not be the first time he has behaved towards his partner in this way.

First, he needs to analyse his sexual behaviour and ask what he expects.

Second, he needs to start seeing an increase in foreplay almost as a personal investment. If he puts in the time, he will reap the reward, not just in his own enhanced pleasure – another common complaint from women is the sexual selfishness of their partners – but in the pleasure that he gives.

And what can the woman do? Men tend to be more simple to please sexually than women. If she examines her own sexual behaviour and finds that she is excluding her partner, the remedy is simple. If her partner likes her to dress and behave to him like a whore or a little-girl-lost from time to time, there is no reason why she should not indulge him. If he likes her to take the lead sometimes, then she should do so.

It is through these sorts of compromises that the foundations for restoring a flagging relationship can be laid and a couple's sex life rejuvenated.

And if a couple have been through this stage once, they will tend to look more closely at their sex life in the future. They will begin to recognize the signs that

indicate sexual boredom is setting in and will be able to take steps to ensure that it is quickly dispelled. In this way a loving couple can get the best out of sex. And a good sex life can go a long way to ensuring that they can overcome any other problems the relationship may encounter.

ORAL LOVEMAKING

Restoring happy and satisfying lovemaking does not suddenly mean that you have to adopt unfamiliar athletic positions or start experimenting with a darker or perverted side of sex. For most couples it means taking what they like best, sexually, and using it in a slightly different way.

Your aim should be to improve the pleasure and quality of orgasms for your partner first, and by so doing enhance your own. What follows are suggestions for adapting your existing lovemaking and for breathing new life into it. All the ideas you will almost certainly have experimented with before – it is just the approach that is different. And if you choose to do something else which you both like, think of ways in which it can be enhanced – good sex takes place more in the mind than anywhere else.

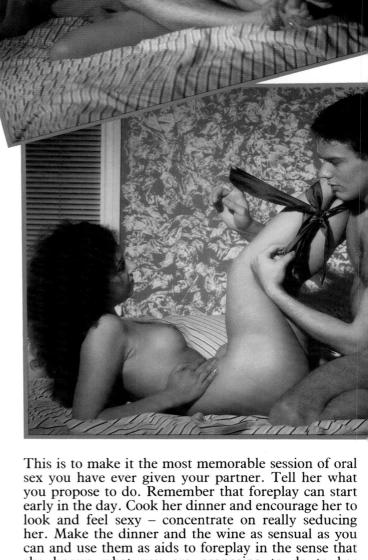

(far right) Making love partially clothed is a great turn-on for many couples and this rear-entry position is ideal for 'quickie' sex

(right) Thinking up new and exciting things to do with each other's bodies can bring a new spice to a couple's lovemaking

ORAL SEX

There are two ways for a couple to use oral sex. They can use it as foreplay before penetration takes place, or they can use it as an alternative form of intercourse. Within these two forms there are a number of variations – the man can perform cunnilingus on the woman, she can fellate him, or they can mutually use their mouths to stimulate each other's genitals – the '69' position.

Whichever way a couple uses it, oral sex can provide exquisite sensations, not only for the recipient, but also for the giver.

The techniques are fairly well chronicled elsewhere, but there are a number of ways that it can be made even more arousing. Here, it is suggested that you use it as a form of intercourse with orgasm taking place – but that is up to you.

FOR HER

Some women believe that men cannot enjoy cunnilingus. They may feel that the genital area is dirty and that the act is somehow unpleasant for the man. Yet, for most men, nothing could be further from the truth. To give pleasure with their lips and tongue and watch the result as they slowly bring their woman to the brink of orgasm and keep her there before she finally surrenders to their lips can be one of the most exciting sexual experiences for a man.

To make the sensations slightly different, it is suggested that the woman remains partially clothes. What she wears is up to her, but it should be whatever makes her feel sexy and whatever her partner likes.

CHOOSE THE PLACE

Varying the place can add a totally new dimension to oral sex. The golden rule should be comfort, however, so if you fancy a change of scene, why not try the settee in the living room or the floor in front of the fire? A few cushions placed strategically around the floor can be both comfortable and arousing.

A little mild bondage can make the sensations even more arousing. If you both like this, use a dressing gown cord or something similar to restrain your partner's arms and legs.

Also, fruit or wine placed in the mouth as you use your tongue on your partner can change the sensations both for you and her.

Whatever you decide to use and wherever you plan to make love, you need to have one idea in your mind.

This is to make it the most memorable session of oral sex you have ever given your partner. Tell her what you propose to do. Remember that foreplay can start early in the day. Cook her dinner and encourage her to look and feel sexy – concentrate on really seducing her. Make the dinner and the wine as sensual as you can and use them as aids to foreplay in the sense that she knows what you are proposing to do to her afterwards. Bath or shower her first – perhaps using oil to massage her. All the time make sure that she knows that she is to be treated specially and that the purpose of all this is to give her an explosive and truly memorable orgasm.

USING YOUR TONGUE

When she is ready, part her legs and use your tongue on the insides of her thighs and her stomach, using a circling motion – spend some time over this. Now, use both hands to part her vaginal lips and – as gently as possible – start to use your tongue around her clitoris, but do not touch it yet.

Use your tongue to trace a path along her perineum and tease her buttocks. Keep the vaginal lips parted and pop your tongue in her vagina, using it as you would your penis. Now, start to use your tongue on her clitoris with a featherlight touch.

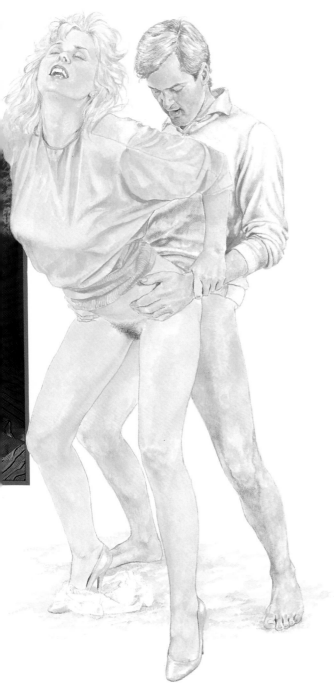

FOR HIM

To give a man a similar experience as you fellate him involves the same type of preparation. The main difference is that because oral sex is so pleasurable to so many men, the chances are that he will come more quickly than you did. Yet, to make the session truly memorable, you need to take some time over it. There are two ways round this. The first is to give him an earlier orgasm so that he is slightly less excited second time around. The other is to squeeze his penis gently as he approaches orgasm. If, of course, your partner has good control then there should be no problems.

The important thing to remember is that, for most men, the longer the orgasm is delayed, the more pleasurable it becomes.

FOREPLAY
Make him dinner and share a bottle of wine. Look sexy for him – if he likes the idea of you wearing no underwear indulge him, but let him know that this is what you have done. After all, for your partner your body is the most stimulating sex aid he knows, so it makes good sex-sense to use it to excite him.

Bath or shower him first and rub some oil into his body, giving him a short sensual massage; but do not touch his penis – massage around it. If he likes being restrained, tie his hands together and also his ankles, and then start to work on his penis with your tongue and lips, slowly increasing the tempo. Use your imagination to increase his pleasure.

WORSHIP HIS PENIS
Keep some clothes on even if it is only some panties or a nightie – whatever he finds most arousing. Tell him what you are going to do and get him to watch. For most men, watching their partner as she takes his penis into her mouth is highly arousing.

Take a comfortable position so that he can see what you are doing and start to lick his penis tip. Run your tongue along the underside of it and perhaps take one of his testicles into your mouth and slowly suck it. Run your tongue along his perineum and then bring it up once more to his penis lip.

Watch him and then take the penis into your mouth and start to suck gently. Keep your hands busy, perhaps sticking a finger gently into his anus as you fellate him. Be guided by his movements and sounds as to how close his orgasm is; when it approaches, grip the root of his penis and squeeze.

As he begins to ejaculate, increase the tempo to its highest pitch and take the semen into your mouth. As he stops thrusting, slow down and lick his penis until his erection subsides.

THE '69' POSITION
Mutual oral sex lends itself to any variety of possibilities. To get the most from a '69' position, it is best if one partner takes control.

Alternate between using your tongue and your teeth and lips in a gentle sucking motions. Pop a couple of fingers into her vagina and use a slow circular motion with your tongue on her clitoris, then start to increase the pace both with fingers and tongue. When she has reached the brink of orgasm withdraw your tongue from her clitoris. Use your fingers perhaps to find her G spot and repeat this several times, always stopping at the verge of orgasm.

Finally, when you sense that she can take no more, use your tongue and lips on her clitoris together with your fingers in her vagina to bring her to orgasm.

Generally, the best positions are those where the woman is on top or if the couple are lying side by side. But if the man can be relied upon to control his thrusting, a good alternative is for the woman to lie back and take the man's penis into her mouth as he thrusts gently into it. As he busies himself using his mouth on her, the increased pressure can provide novel sensations for both partners.

VARIETY

Part of the reason that sex becomes routine is that each partner knows exactly what to expect from the other. There is nothing wrong with this but familiarity is a double-edged sword. It provides the best sex because a couple know what the other likes best, but it also discourages experimenting with unknown positions – which is one of the reasons that an otherwise satisfactory sex life can start to flag and deteriorate.

ADAPTING FAVOURED POSITIONS
The problem is further compounded by the fact that a couple come to know after a period what they like best sexually – they discover this by trial and error. So a favourite position or technique – used again and again – can be seen as one of the causes of declining sexually when, in fact, it is nothing of the sort.

A couple probably do not need new positions – especially if they have already tried and tested them – but they may need to approach the favoured ones in a slightly different way or even in a different or unusual setting.

This is simpler than it sounds. If you have been making love regularly at the same time on the same nights each week, it is a simple matter to change your habits. Simply vary the time and place – any room in the house can be as conducive to lovemaking as can any time of the day.

In this position the man has to partially support his partner by holding her buttocks as he pushes her against the wall. It is only really suitable for lovers who have a good deal of stamina

And for the couple who want to add a little extra to their lovemaking, making love half-clothed and in a hurry may be just what they need from time to time.

HIM – TO HER

Surprise lovemaking for your partner may be a real turn-on, the main reason being that it shows that you find her so desirable that you cannot resist her. And being partially or even fully clothed can bring back that frenetic excitement of when you made love to each other for the first time.

For the purposes of 'surprise lovemaking', it is essential that the woman is wearing a skirt that can be easily lifted up. Do not, however, attempt intercourse straight away. Kiss and caress your partner until she is aroused, but instead of making love to her on the bed, make love to her standing up – rear-entry lovemaking is probably the most suitable position for this.

Turn her round so that she is facing a wall and get her to press her hands against it. Lift up her skirt and remove her panties and enter her. Use your hands to stimulate her clitoris and try to bring her to orgasm.

HER – TO HIM

Most men are receptive to the idea of surprise lovemaking – it flatters them that their partner wants them so desperately that she cannot wait. However, you cannot rely on him having an instant erection so – when the time is right – you will have to arouse him in some way – either manually or orally.

When his penis is erect, put your arms round his neck and take him over to a wall where your back can be supported. Jump up on him and get him to enter you. Use the wall to apply pressure so that you can move your buttocks as freely as possible. Most of the thrusting will come from you as you 'bounce' up and down on his penis.

OTHER IDEAS
These are only two suggestions. Almost any position can be adapted in this way. It is not recommended as the type of lovemaking that a couple should use all the time, but as an occasional sexual adventure it should do much to restore interest to an otherwise routine sex life. Also, thinking up your own ideas on how to vary your sex life will greatly increase your level of arousal.

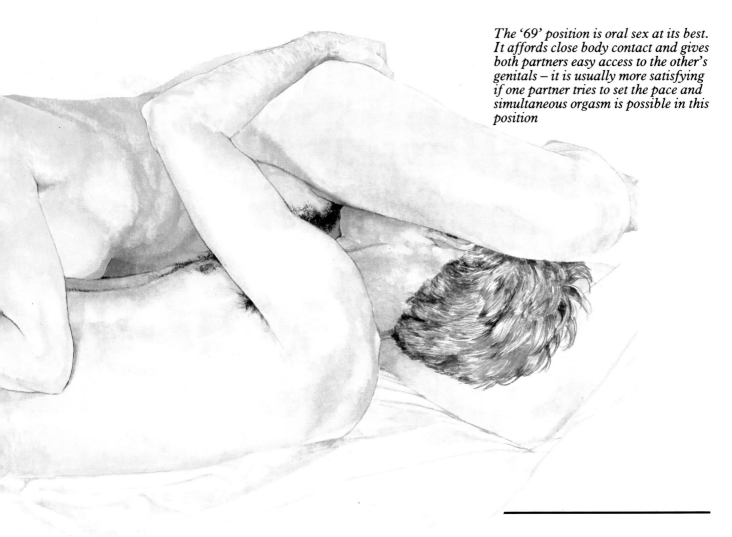

The '69' position is oral sex at its best. It affords close body contact and gives both partners easy access to the other's genitals – it is usually more satisfying if one partner tries to set the pace and simultaneous orgasm is possible in this position

A LIFETIME
OF LOVING

From puberty onwards, most of us make love more times than we can remember. And, although the quantity may decline over the years, the quality of sex can be greatly enhanced as we grow into middle age and beyond. All that is needed is a little imagination, an open mind – and a loving and considerate partner

Our potential for sexual and erotic pleasure begins when we are born and does not end – or need not end – until we die. Yet, during our lives, the quality and quantity of our sexual responses and experiences are affected by the changes involved in the ageing process.

MALE AND FEMALE RESPONSES
Two major studies of sexuality – those of Kinsey, and Masters and Johnson – both concluded that men reach their sexual peak around the age of 18 and start to deteriorate afterwards. Women reach their sexual peak in their thirties, or even forties, and thereafter decline at a slower rate than men. So the main problem that a couple have to contend with as they age is that the man reaches his sexual peak some 15 or 20 years earlier than the woman. Yet orgasm is common to both sexes and can be experienced even into old age.

EARLY MALE SEXUALITY
Infant boys have erections and handle their genitals from birth and continue to do so throughout infancy. At puberty, a boy starts to experience a sudden and dramatic change in his sexuality.

After his first ejaculation, he starts to experience an urgency for orgasms; and sexual desire enters – and may even dominate – his life. At no other point in his life will he be able to reach orgasm as quickly or as often as he does during these early years.

Fantasies and dreams become more and more explicit and erotic and the adolescent male starts to look for sexual partners. If no partner is available, he will almost certainly masturbate himself regularly to orgasm. If he does not masturbate or seek some other outlet, he will almost certainly have nocturnal emissions – wet dreams.

In these early years, a boy's interest in sex will

TEENS

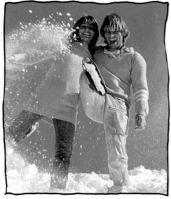

A time for learning and discovery – and confusion – as adolescent boys and girls become aware of their growing sexuality and begin the search for sexual partners

TWENTIES

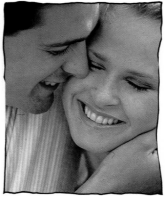

Now that they are more at ease with their sexuality, both sexes start to experiment and explore each other – usually within the framework of a stable relationship

THIRTIES

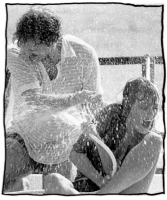

Although the man is on the sexual decline in terms of frequency of orgasms, he can compensate for this with better control. The woman is now at her most orgasmic

tend to outweigh his ability to find partners – in the United Kingdom roughly 50 per cent of males do not have their first experience of full sexual intercourse until they are aged 19.

It is ironic that this point in his life where he experiences his peak of sexual desire coincides with a period where he probably finds sexual partners most difficult to find. However, although his sexual technique will be primitive, it is probably fair to say that at no time in his life will he find sex quite so exciting and stimulating.

EARLY FEMALE SEXUALITY

Unlike an adolescent boy, a girl is not at her most orgasmic by the time she has completed puberty. At the same stage, girls also undergo a dramatic increase in their sex drive, but they probably tend to be more concerned with attracting boys rather than have sex with them.

And although a girl may have intercourse with a partner, she is less likely to have an orgasm than he is. This is partly because a boy of the same age will find his orgasm difficult to regulate, will probably spend too little time on foreplay, and also because she is still several years away from her sexual peak.

One study of female sexuality shows that, at puberty, only one-fifth of girls have orgasms. By the early twenties this will have risen to around 75 per cent and it will not peak until the thirties and forties, where the figure for women's orgasms then hovers around 90 per cent.

TWENTIES

A man in his twenties continues to want sexual release at much the same frequency as he did in puberty, even though he is already on the sexual decline. According to Kinsey, four to eight orgasms a day at this stage are still not uncommon.

Partners will be more available than they were in his teenage years and, as he starts to have intercourse with a regular partner, he will learn to delay his own orgasm and lengthen the duration of intercourse.

The frequency with which a couple have intercourse together reaches a peak at this stage.

Yet, although the experience of intercourse is frequent, the woman has still to attain her own sexual peak. The quality of sex may have improved for her at this stage, certainly if she is making love regularly to her partner, but she is not yet at her most orgasmic. She will also require more foreplay than her male counterpart of the same age.

THIRTIES AND FORTIES

The number of times he achieves orgasm becomes less important to a man during his thirties.

He will still be extremely interested in sex – that is unlikely to waver for some years yet – but he will be less preoccupied with the frequency of his own orgasms. One or two should serve to satisfy him during each bout of lovemaking.

He will still obtain erections regularly, but he is unlikely to ejaculate as frequently as he used to, unless the conditions are unusually conducive – perhaps during an affair or if the circumstances with his regular partner are unusually stimulating.

His ability to control his own orgasms – perhaps because they are less frequent and therefore more precious, but also because he is more experienced – should be more marked at this age.

By the time he reaches his forties, the quality of his

FORTIES

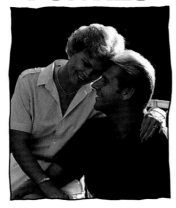

For most men, the raw urgency of youth has been replaced with more sensuality and consideration. The woman is still at the height of her sexual potential

FIFTIES

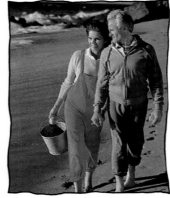

Quantity of sex is now less important and is replaced with a gentler, more subtle approach. Free from birth control worries, a couple can enjoy unhibited lovemaking

SIXTIES
and beyond.

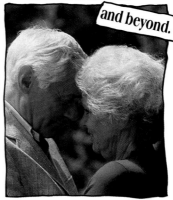

The experience of age and the contentment of a lifetime together both help to ensure that sex remains a unique, shared experience between two long-term lovers

sexual pleasure will have noticeably changed from the intense urgency of youth to a less frequent, but more sensuous and appreciative experience, which will continue into later life. Orgasm will become less important to him.

All this is in complete contrast to the woman of the same age. Most women reach their peak of sexuality in their thirties and forties. Masters and Johnson observed a much more ready response in women, especially after the birth of several children. They also found that vaginal lubrication occurs much more quickly, possibly decreasing the amount of foreplay necessary to bring them to orgasm.

Accompanying her increased physiological responses probably comes a shedding of earlier psychological inhibitions and a familiarity with her partner who now knows what she likes best sexually.

FIFTIES AND SIXTIES

From about the age of 40, a man's testes become less efficient at producing sperm and the hormone testosterone. This results in a decrease in the firmness and size of the testicles, greater difficulty in obtaining an erection and fewer ejaculations. There will almost certainly be an increase in the length of time between ejaculations as well.

However, the resultant sexual decline is very gradual and extends over a long period – perhaps 20 or 30 years.

There is no set pattern for a woman and her sex life as she reaches middle age. Statistically, the years between 35 and 50 are when she is at her most orgasmic, but this is her physical capability on a variety of factors.

Most women recognize that their sexual desires change according to their lifestyle, work, the time of the month and any of the commitment that they may have. And most recognize, as well, that sex will continue to be as satisfactory as it was in their middle twenties – perhaps even more so.

Once the hormonal imbalance of the menopause is restored, women can often look forward to a new life, free from worries about birth control, pregnancy and all the associated discomforts. Many women find that their sex lives actually improve and that now they can concentrate purely on their own needs and those of their partner.

For both men and women, there is no reason why sex should not continue to be satisfying and fulfilling.

TIME TO TALK

If everyone started making love every day at puberty and continued until they were 80, they would have made love more than 22,000 times.

For most people, the amount of times will be considerably less, and will be determined by many factors – their sex drive, what sort of person they are, how often they fall in love, whether they marry, whether they become seriously ill and so on.

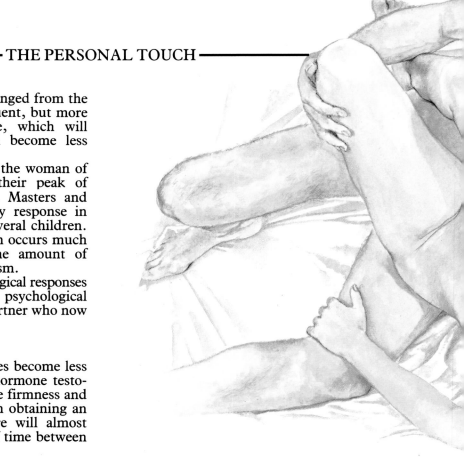

Even if a person were to remain free of the sexual, emotional and psychological events that make our lives, no sexual relationship is, or ever could be, totally static – no-one would wish it this way.

Sexual appetites vary from person to person and couple to couple. And there will be times in every person's life when they are more sexually active than at others, usually in stress-free periods.

The quantity, as well as the quality, of the sex we experience varies throughout our lives. Clinical experience has shown, however, that some sexual positions are particularly suitable for the needs and desires of specific age groups. Their main aim is to compensate for the 'imbalance' of sexual needs which affects the sexes at different ages.

18-29

This is a time of experimentation for both sexes. Sex is usually frequent although sexual difficulties arising out of inexperience are common.

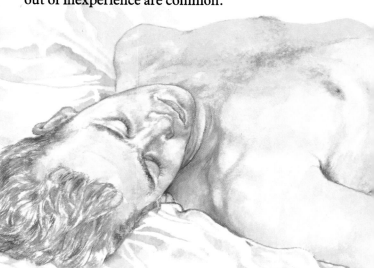

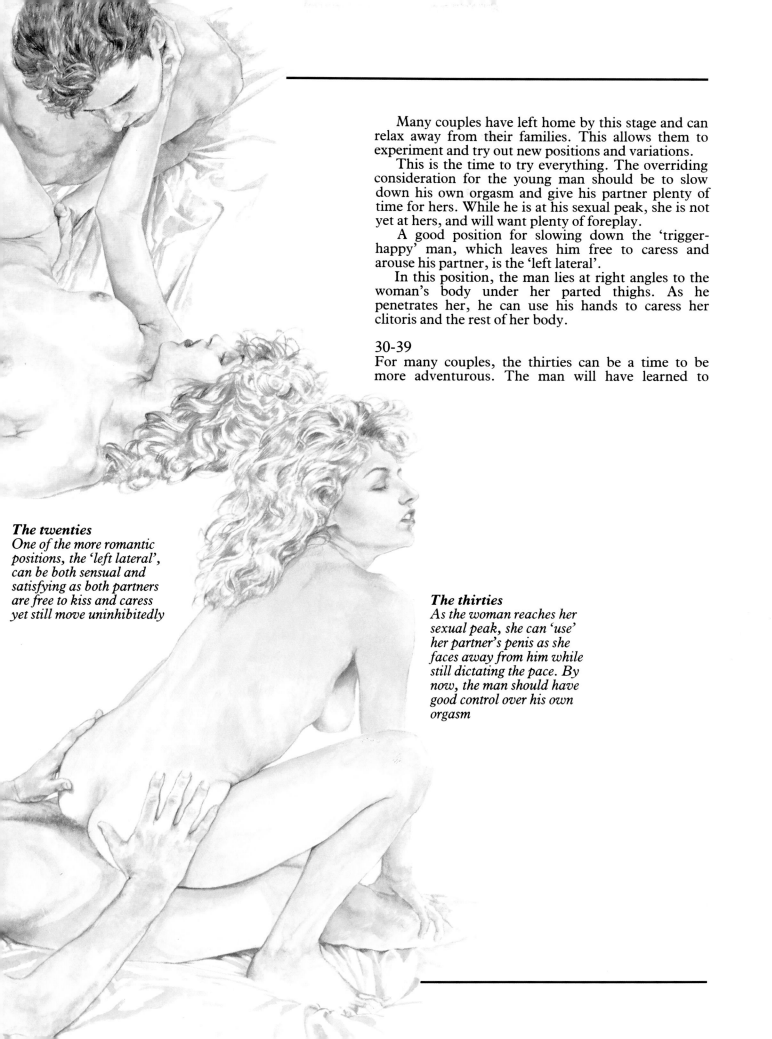

Many couples have left home by this stage and can relax away from their families. This allows them to experiment and try out new positions and variations.

This is the time to try everything. The overriding consideration for the young man should be to slow down his own orgasm and give his partner plenty of time for hers. While he is at his sexual peak, she is not yet at hers, and will want plenty of foreplay.

A good position for slowing down the 'trigger-happy' man, which leaves him free to caress and arouse his partner, is the 'left lateral'.

In this position, the man lies at right angles to the woman's body under her parted thighs. As he penetrates her, he can use his hands to caress her clitoris and the rest of her body.

30-39
For many couples, the thirties can be a time to be more adventurous. The man will have learned to

The twenties
One of the more romantic positions, the 'left lateral', can be both sensual and satisfying as both partners are free to kiss and caress yet still move uninhibitedly

The thirties
As the woman reaches her sexual peak, she can 'use' her partner's penis as she faces away from him while still dictating the pace. By now, the man should have good control over his own orgasm

control his orgasm, although he may not come as frequently as he did in his twenties. The woman is beginning the most orgasmic period of her life.

She now often has the experience and confidence to take charge from time to time, so as to please herself. Any of the woman-on-top positions allow her to control the pace and tempo of lovemaking.

Facing away from her partner, particularly, enables her to 'use' him in an unhibited and abandoned way.

40-49

The man's sexual powers may start to diminish in his forties even though his partner is still potentially highly orgasmic. To offset this, she may need to increase the quality and quantity of the stimulation she gives him.

All the lessons of foreplay learned earlier in a couple's life can be used at this time – oral sex may well be particularly satisfying for him. The man can continue to arouse his woman, of course, and by so doing will arouse himself.

For a man – or woman – who has fantasies of anal sex, rear-entry positions, where the woman is penetrated from behind, are greatly enjoyable.

50-59

The 'missionary' position can be particularly well suited to couples in this age group; indeed, it will probably have been used throughout a great deal of their lives together.

Really deep penetration could be painful or uncomfortable after the woman's menopause, so it makes good sense to go for shallow positions such as the 'missionary'.

60 AND BEYOND

Now is the time for romantic rather than athletic positions. Sexual desire, and the need to give and receive physical love, is still strong – but older bodies are, of course, less agile.

The man can try kneeling in front of the woman as she lies on a bed or low table with her legs apart as he enters her.

GOLDEN RULES

The truly loving couple will vary their sexual activity throughout their sexual lives together. Finding and experimenting with different positions is only one part of their joint sex life. As they age, there are lessons that most partners forget and would, perhaps, do well to remember.

☐ Make sure that you have plenty of physical contact. Kissing and cuddling are part of loveplay, but they can also be an end in themselves.

☐ Treat your partner as you would like to be treated – do as you would be done by. All of us are susceptible to presents and compliments, and too often we think things and do not say them. Any time in a relationship is a good time to start doing this.

☐ Talk to each other. This is probably the most

NO AGE LIMITS

As a couple grow older, the frequency with which they make love does not decline as much as popular myth would have it.

Between the ages of 25 and 55 or beyond, the frequency with which couples have intercourse gradually declines from three times a week to only once a week on average.

These figures probablty over-emphasize the fall-off, because people in younger age groups tend to change partners more than older men and women (and most people make love more frequently at the start of a relationship).

The forties
Rear-entry positions allow deep penetration which should be both satisfying for the woman and stimulating for the man – particularly if the couple share fantasies about anal sex

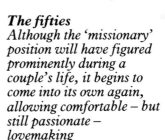

The fifties
Although the 'missionary' position will have figured prominently during a couple's life, it begins to come into its own again, allowing comfortable – but still passionate – lovemaking

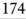

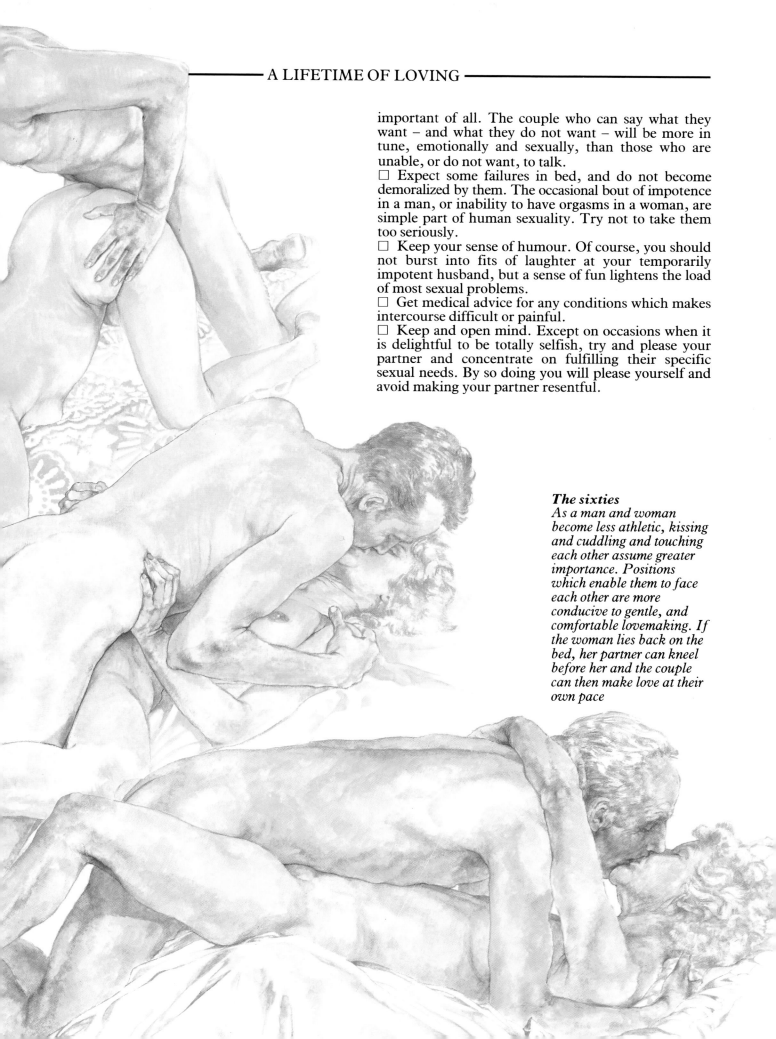

important of all. The couple who can say what they want – and what they do not want – will be more in tune, emotionally and sexually, than those who are unable, or do not want, to talk.

☐ Expect some failures in bed, and do not become demoralized by them. The occasional bout of impotence in a man, or inability to have orgasms in a woman, are simple part of human sexuality. Try not to take them too seriously.

☐ Keep your sense of humour. Of course, you should not burst into fits of laughter at your temporarily impotent husband, but a sense of fun lightens the load of most sexual problems.

☐ Get medical advice for any conditions which makes intercourse difficult or painful.

☐ Keep and open mind. Except on occasions when it is delightful to be totally selfish, try and please your partner and concentrate on fulfilling their specific sexual needs. By so doing you will please yourself and avoid making your partner resentful.

The sixties
As a man and woman become less athletic, kissing and cuddling and touching each other assume greater importance. Positions which enable them to face each other are more conducive to gentle, and comfortable lovemaking. If the woman lies back on the bed, her partner can kneel before her and the couple can then make love at their own pace

CONTRACEPTION

Despite the availability of family planning and an increasing range of contraceptives, millions of women throughout the world still risk unplanned pregnancy because they and their partners do not use regular or reliable contraception

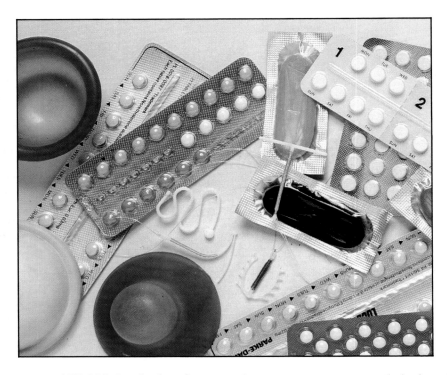

In 1989 there were over 187,000 legal abortions performed in the UK; this figure does not differ much from year to year, and the number of unintended pregnancies remains stubbornly high.

One reason is that information about contraception is often not reaching the people that most need it. As a result, couples and individuals often make the wrong decisions about the methods they choose, use them badly, or abandon them altogether. Others are not using contraception at all and simply taking a chance that they do not get pregnant.

This is not really surprising since information about contraceptive methods is changing all the time. As methods are tested and researched, more risks and side effects come to light and the more confusing it all becomes – for doctors as well as the consumers.

Choice becomes even more complicated as scientific research points to limiting medical methods of contraception to particular ages and groups of women.

At the same time women have learned to understand and appreciate their bodies far more and are less inclined simply to accept what they are prescribed. Increasingly, they are attracted by methods which they see as more natural, in keeping with the general trend towards a more natural lifestyle.

SHARING THE CHOICE

With the arrival of the Pill and IUD (Intra-Uterine Device) in the 1960s, women took responsibility for contraception and were relieved to have the means of preventing pregnancy under their own control. But many women now feel resentful that they shoulder all the risks and problems, while more men feel unhappy that they have no role to play.

Time and time again, studies show that men's intentions in terms of sharing responsibility for contraception are often very positive. Unfortunately, these same studies show that for most men there is a wide gap between intention and practice.

There is no ideal contraceptive, nor is there likely to be for decades. But good methods do exist. They all have advantages and disadvantges, and the way individuals or couples assess these very much depends on their lifestyle and attitudes to sex.

For many people there will be a different 'best method' at different times of their life. For couples the

CONTRACEPTIVE METHODS AND EFFECTIVENESS	
Information from leaflets and Fact Sheets published by the UK Family Planning Information Service (May 1991)	
METHOD	**EFFECTIVENESS**
THE COMBINED PILL (triphasic and biphasic pills/Everyday Pill)	99% (if taken properly)
MINI-PILL	99% (if taken properly)
INJECTABLE CONTRACEPTIVES (Depo-Provera/Noristerat)	Over 99%
IUD	97–99%
DIAPHRAGM or CAP (plus spermicide)	85–98% (with careful use)
SPONGE	75–91% (with careful use)
SHEATH	85–98% (with careful use)
'SAFE PERIOD' (body-temperature method)	80–98% (with careful use)
FEMALE STERILIZATION	Occasional failure: 1 in 200–1 in 1,000*
MALE STERILIZATION	Occasional failure: 1 in 1,000
Effectiveness rates for reversible methods refer to the number of women out of 100 using the method for a year who do not get pregnant. Post-coital effectiveness	rates refer to the number of women out of 100 who do not become pregnant after using post-coital methods. * Depending on method used.

solution to sharing the responsibility may be to alternate between male and female methods.

Doctors and nurses can help you make a choice, and counselling services are gradually becoming more accessible to men as well as women, but in the end the decision has to be yours. A good choice of contraceptive can help you enjoy a relaxed sex life as well as protecting against unintended pregnancy.

THE PILL

When most people refer to the Pill, they mean the oral contraceptive which contains two hormones, oestrogen and progestogen, that stop women ovulating.

The Pill became available in the early 1960s and it gained popularity, after initial problems, to become the most used method of birth control and almost synonymous with contraception. But in the last 25 or so years a great deal of information has been collected on the effects of the Pill on women's health.

Some of this information is inconclusive and confusing, but it has resulted in more thought being given to minimizing side effects and the production of a second generation of contraceptive Pills which contained much lower doses of hormones.

THE PILL AND THE RISKS

To some extent it has also become possible to identify these women who might run risks from taking the Pill, such as smokers, those who are overweight or those with high blood pressure.

Since the publication of reports in October 1983, suggesting possible, but unconfirmed, links between taking the Pill and breast and cervical cancer, women are increasingly questioning that crucial balance between reliability and safety.

The great attraction of the Pill has always been its reliability together with its convenience. For many

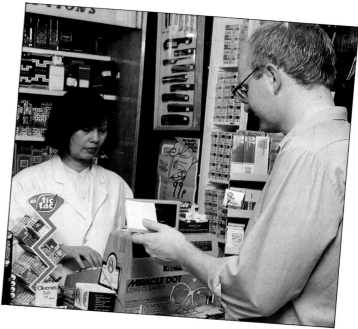

Sheaths, the only contraceptive product available for men, can be bought readily from any chemist

couples the Pill is the only method which allows them to be completely spontaneous in their lovemaking.

Many women are trying to weigh up the plusses and minuses of taking the Pill. The most serious condition linked with the Pill is thrombosis, although the risk is very small unless you smoke or are overweight. Other side effects include depression, weight gain, loss of sex drive and headaches, although these can often be stopped by changing to a different Pill. It is worth remembering, however, that the Pill may protect against some diseases such as cancer of the ovaries and rheumatoid arthritis. And it is certainly the most convenient form of contraception at present.

THE MINI-PILL

For some women looking to minimize the health risks of Pill-taking, a move to the mini-Pill will provide a good solution. Mini-Pills contain only one hormone, progestogen, and the dose is lower than the progestogen dose in the combined Pill. They do not stop ovulation but prevent pregnancy in other ways, such as thickening the mucus at the entrance to the cervix to make it difficult for the sperm to penetrate.

As it does not contain oestrogen the mini-Pill is not thought to contribute to the risks of thrombosis, not have mini-Pills been implicated in the recent cancer scares. On the other hand, they are less effective, and if a pregnancy does happen there is some risk of it being outside the womb – most probably in the Fallopian tubes. Women taking the mini-Pill also tend to suffer from irregular, or break-through, bleeding.

Mini-Pills must be taken every day at exactly the same time each day to be effective. They are usually considered most suitable for older women and breast-feeding mothers, but are not yet widely prescribed.

LONGER-ACTING METHODS

Depo-provera is a synthetic progestogen which is given by injection, usually into the muscle of the buttock. It is absorbed over a period of three months and stops ovulation.

Use of Depo-provera as a contraceptive has been controversial, and for many years it was only licensed in Britain for short-term use in special circumstances. In 1984, however, it was given a licence for long-term use and is slowly becoming more readily available.

The controversy has arisen partly because of unpleasant side effects such as irregular and frequent bleeding, weight gain and delays in return of fertility, and partly because of unsubstantiated fears of breast cancer and cancer of the lining of the womb.

There is concern that Depo-provera is sometimes given without proper explanation, so that women are

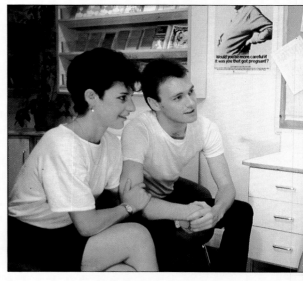

A chat with a counsellor to discuss the various methods may make the final decision easier

misled about possible side effects and sometimes suffer badly until the effect of the drug wears off.

The advantages of Depo-provera are its high reliability and ease of use. Most family planning experts, however, do not see it as a first-choice method of contraceptive, but rather as a useful addition to the range of contraceptives suitable for those unable to use other methods.

There is another injectable hormone called Noris-terat now available, which lasts for two months and is used as an extra precaution after a vasectomy.

IUD, OR COIL

An Intra-Uterine Device (IUD) is a small 2.5cm (1in)-long flexible plastic device, now usually wound with copper, which is inserted into the womb by a doctor.

Coils come in a variety of different shapes and are

MALE PILLS AND OTHER MALE METHODS

Today, new possibilities for contraception lie in the development of a male Pill.

Magazine surveys show that men have a variety of reactions to the idea of shouldering the responsibility of contraception by taking a pill every day.

Women, too, while wanting to shift the responsibility, question how dedicated men would be in taking it regularly. After all, it is not the man who gets pregnant if he forgets to take it.

A male Pill is actually more difficult to 'design' than the female Pill beause there is no single event – like the release of the female egg – on which to work.

The most promising male Pill so far has come from China and was discovered by accident when it was noticed that in rural areas, where cotton-seed oil was used for cooking, the men had become infertile.

The first clinical trials on the plant extract gossypol, responsible for the infertility, started in China in 1972 and were reported six years later. The results were very encouraging, the effectiveness was nearly 100 per cent and there were few side effects.

Further research carried out by the World Health Organisation (but which has been abandoned) showed that side

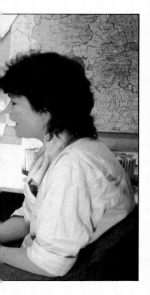

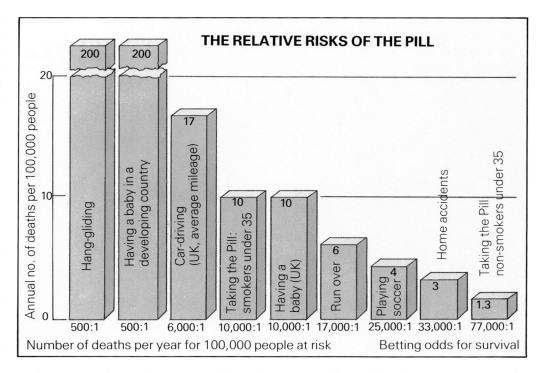

THE RELATIVE RISKS OF THE PILL

Annual no. of deaths per 100,000 people

| 200 | 200 | 17 | 10 | 10 | 6 | 4 | 3 | 1.3 |

- Hang-gliding
- Having a baby in a developing country
- Car-driving (UK, average mileage)
- Taking the Pill: smokers under 35
- Having a baby (UK)
- Run over
- Playing soccer
- Home accidents
- Taking the Pill: non-smokers under 35

| 500:1 | 500:1 | 6,000:1 | 10,000:1 | 10,000:1 | 17,000:1 | 25,000:1 | 33,000:1 | 77,000:1 |

Number of deaths per year for 100,000 people at risk   Betting odds for survival

normally replaced every two to five years, depending on the type. Although no one knows exactly how an IUD works, it prevents an egg from implanting in the womb lining.

Like the Pill, the coil was introduced in the 1960s, but has never achieved the same popularity. One reasons for this was that early coils were not usually a first choice for women who had not had a child, for they were rather large in relation to the size of the womb.

More recently, copper-wound coils are smaller, but now there are different reasons why these are not recommended to women who have not had children. The problem is that the presence of a coil makes a woman more susceptible to pelvic infection which can be difficult to deal with and which could affect her ability to conceive later on.

The failure rate of the coil is about the same as the mini-Pill and, like the mini-Pill, pregnancies that do occur could be ectopic (occuring outside the womb).

One of its main disadvantages is that it often causes heavier periods. There may also be bleeding between periods. One of the main advantages is that, once fitted, there is no further involvement by the woman, except to check now and then that it is in the correct place by feeling the threads. An internal check-up by your doctor every year or so is essential.

BARRIER METHODS

Men and women started using barriers of various kinds to prevent pregnancy thousands of years ago.

Currently available are the diaphragm, cervical cap, vault cap and vimule cap. They are all made of soft rubber and fit over the neck of the womb.

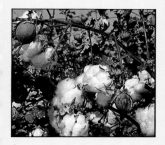

effects were more common than first thought, including feeling weak, digestive problems and loss of sex drive.

The conclusion seems to be that gossypol itself will not be the male Pill of the future, but something similar instead.

Other Pills could be developed from existing drugs, such as one used for hypertension. This particular drug acts as an 'ejaculation inhibitor'.

Also being researched is the injection of the synthetic hormone – 19-nortestosterone which is used by some athletes to build up their muscles Unfortunately, however, the drug has the strange side effect of reducing the testicles to half their normal size.

A mixture of the hormones oestradiol and testosterone rubbed into the abdomen has been unsuccessful, as in trials it caused men's partners to grow moustaches

A male version of the 'releasing' hormone nasal spray and a mix of hormone introduced by a tiny pump have had no success so far.

INTRA-UTERINE DEVICES (IUDs) AND BARRIER METHODS

THE CHOICE:
IUDs (and applicator), the sponge, diaphragm, vault cap and cervical cap

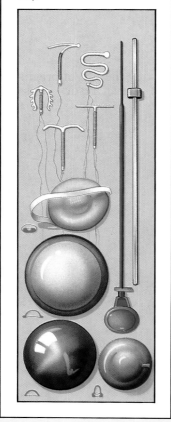

FITTING AN IUD (COIL)

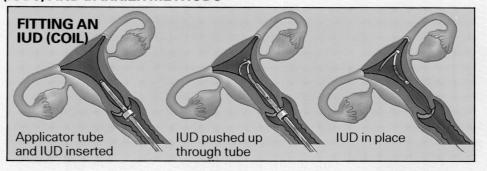

Applicator tube and IUD inserted

IUD pushed up through tube

IUD in place

The IUD is fitted by a doctor. It is threaded into an applicator, which is inserted into the vagina and through the cervical opening. The IUD is passed through the applicator tube into the womb

Diaphragms and caps must be used with a spermicide, and initially fitted by a doctor or nurse, who gives instructions on how to use them. The contraceptive sponge works on similar principles

APPROXIMATE POSITION OF DIAPHRAGM OR CAP

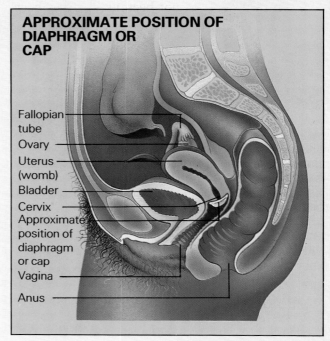

Fallopian tube
Ovary
Uterus (womb)
Bladder
Cervix
Approximate position of diaphragm or cap
Vagina
Anus

They are used with spermicide cream or jelly, and inserted before lovemaking to form a barrier to sperm.

The newest barrier is the contraceptive sponge. Even though it is less reliable than the diaphragm, and therefore only suitable for women for whom pregnancy would not be disastrous, it overcomes some of the main objects to diaphragms and caps.

A major complaint by women is that barrier methods are too messy, interfere with spontaneous lovemaking and look unattractive. The sponge which is left in place for at least six hours after sex, is impregnated with spermicide and after one use thrown away.

The male sheath is making a comeback. It is a reliable barrier method which rarely has any side effects. Today's sheaths are finer than ever before and often ribbed for increased sensation.

'SAFE PERIOD' METHODS

These are usually used by couples who have objections to other methods for religious or other reasons. They are becoming increasingly popular with women who do not want to use medical or mechanical methods to avoid pregnancy. And as women become more aware of changes throughout their reproductive cycle, they are drawn to methods they are finely tuned to their own needs.

'Safe period' methods aim to pinpoint when a woman is most fertile and to avoid intercourse at this time. She will have to note signs of ovulation by taking her temperature every day (body-temperature method) or examining her cervical mucus (Billings method).

Careful record-keeping is essential, as is high motivation by both partners, with the acceptance that there will be times when they cannot have intercourse. These methods do need to be learned and are not suitable for women with irregular periods or for a while after childbirth, as absolute accuracy is vital for predicting 'safe-periods'.

'Safe period' methods do not give the reliability that most couples demand. The effectiveness is increased when the temperature method is combined with the Billings method and other signs of ovulation, but the failure rate is still high.

Most people have heard about the 'morning-after' Pill, but fewer know about the post-coital IUD, which is another option.

The post-coital Pill is in fact a special dose of the contraceptive Pill containing oestrogen and progestogen, which is taken within 72 hours of intercourse. The fitting of a coil within five days after intercourse is the alternative.

Morning-after methods have become generally available and endorsed for safety in recent years. They are, it should be stressed, only for use in an emergency – when contraception has not been used or has been used but has failed.

The post-coital Pill method involves taking a special dose of hormones under a doctor's supervision. However, it will only work for the one occasion. Sometimes side effects such as nausea, and occasionally vomiting, are experienced. Once fitted, the post-coital coil will ensure continuous protection.

STERILIZATION

Female sterilization and male vasectomy are intended as permanent methods of birth control. They involve relatively simply operations that close the Fallopian tubes in a woman, and the tubes through which sperm travels in a man.

A vasectomy is usually done under local anaesthetic and takes a few minutes. Female sterilization takes longer and can be done under general or local anaesthetic.

There are several ways female sterilization can be carried out, the most common being by laparoscopy when the Fallopian tubes are blocked with rings or clips. Neither the male nor female operation affects the production of hormones responsible for sexual drive, so sexual feelings should not be changed, unless they are improved by removing the risk of pregnancy.

Sterilization was once a last resort chosen by couples who had had many children. Today, it is increasingly chosen by couples who have decided that they have completed their family. In many countries one in five women in the fertile age range have been sterilized or their partners have had a vasectomy. It is seen nowadays as a positive and responsible step.

However, in a time of increasing marriage breakdown, there are also more requests for reversal. But reversal operations are frequently not effective, so sterilization operations really should be regarded as permanent and irreversible.

THE 'SAFE PERIOD' METHODS

The principle of safe period methods of contraception is to learn to predict and recognize the time of the month when you are most fertile, and to avoid intercourse at that time. Sex is thus restricted to 'safe' days, when you are less likely to conceive.

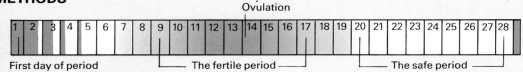

Ovulation

First day of period — The fertile period — The safe period

A woman is most likely to get pregnant at and around the time of ovulation – when the egg is released from the ovary into the Fallopian tube. This usually occurs about two weeks before the start of the next period, but there are various ways that a woman can pin-point the precise moment more accurately.

Since sperm can live for up to five days inside a woman, and an egg can live for about two days, a woman must not have sex for at least five days before ovulation and for several days afterwards. Calculating the time of ovulation (when sex should be avoided) can be done in several ways:
☐ The body-temperature method
☐ The Billings (mucus) method
☐ The calendar method
☐ Combinations of these methods

The body-temperature method The woman takes her temperature every morning on waking up, and keeps a special chart. Immediately before ovulation, body temperature drops slightly – after the egg is released, it rises to a higher level than in the previous week.

The Billings (mucus) method This method works on the principle that ovulation can be detected by changes in cervical mucus. The woman is taught to examine her mucus and to recognize changes – such as increased amount and 'wetness'.

The calendar method The woman is shown how to calculate when she is most likely to ovulate by keeping a long-term record of her menstrual cycle. On its own this method is *very* unreliable and is not recommended.

Combined methods Combining methods and learning to recognize other 'symptoms' of ovulation increases the reliability. With all these natural methods, skilled guidance is essential. See your doctor or family planning clinic for advice.

These techniques are most successful for women who have regular periods. Anything which makes periods irregular – from the recent birth of a baby to a change of routine – makes ovulation difficult to predict. Pain-killing drugs can alter body temperature and make the temperature method rather unreliable.

SEXUAL DISEASES

Sexually transmitted diseases are on the increase throughout the world, and young people form a high proportion of those affected. But if diagnosed early some of these infections can be cured

Any disease that can be passed on from one person to another by sexual contact is called a sexually transmitted disease, or STD. In the past the term VD (short for veneral disease) was much more commonly used, and usually referred to gonorrhoea and syphilis, the more serious of the diseases, apart from the killer disease AIDS, which is discussed fully later in the book.

For many people, VD was not merely a term describing an infectious disease transmitted sexually – it was regarded as something that was only caught by people who indulged in immoral behaviour. This attitude has changed a great deal in recent years, so that today STDs, and departments of genito-urinary medicine where they are treated, are usually thought of with less embarrassment than in the past.

WHO SUFFERS?
Anyone can catch an STD by oral and anal sex as well as by vaginal intercourse; in most cases the treatment for the infection is not painful or difficult. However, the earlier it is diagnosed, the easier it is to cure.

Generally, the most severe consequences of neglected STD fall upon women and babies. Women are far less likely to have the recognizable symptoms that make early diagnosis easy. That is why the follow-up of contacts by an STD clinic is so important.

Not surprisingly, some 60 per cent of those infected worldwide are under 24. The effect on young women can be particularly devastating if the untreated disease leads to infertility. So, if you think you could have caught an infection, even though you have no symptoms, go for a check-up anyway – nobody is going to criticize you for being safe rather than sorry, and it is better to put your mind at rest.

SYPHILIS
Syphilis, one of the most serious of all STDs, is becoming less common in Great Britain and the western world generally, while increasing in the developing world. There are about 20 to 50 million cases in the world every year. There were around 1,300 cases reported in Great Britain in 1989, over 21 per cent fewer than in 1987 – with around twice as many men as women contracting the disease.

WHAT IS SYPHILIS?
Syphilis is caused by a corkscrew-shaped organism which is present in the blood and body fluids of an infected person. It can only live in the warm environment that the body provides. The likelihood of you contracting syphilis if you have sex with an infected person is though to be about one in two – particularly when it is in the early stages.

When the disease is passed on (by contact with a sore or ulcer), minute organisms, called triponemes, pass through the skin. After only half an hour they have passed to the lymph nodes in the groin and next they pass into the blood stream and are distributed to the whole body. In about three weeks, the body's defence mechanism begins to work against them.

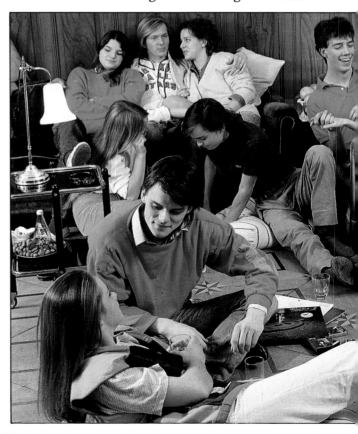

THE FIRST SYMPTOMS

The first symptoms of syphilis is a raised pimple on the vagina or penis (although it can sometimes occur on the mouth or anus from or oral or anal contact).

Next, hard tissue forms around the pimple. The pimple becomes a painless ulcer or sore from which fluid oozes, and finally heals leaving a scar, usually taking about three weeks to do so.

Most people seek treatment when the sore appears; the doctor will take a sample of the fluid from the sore to examine under a microscope and will also look to see if the lymph nodes of the groin are swollen.

The doctor will also take blood tests to see if antibodies to the organisms have been manufactured by the blood.

EFFECTS ON THE UNBORN CHILD

Transmission of syphilis to an unborn baby occurs by way of the placenta. A blood test done, for example, in the first ten weeks of pregnancy, can diagnose the disease in the mother before it is passed on to the baby – which does not happen until after the twentieth week. She can be cured with penicillin and produce a perfectly healthy baby.

TREATMENT

The chances of curing early syphilis by penicillin or other antibiotics are excellent, and even the advanced disease can be arrested. Daily injections of penicillin (together with Probenecid which maintains high levels of the antibiotic in the bloodstream) are given for about ten days, or a single dose can be injected into a muscle. Alternative antibiotics are given to those allergic to penicillin.

GONORRHOEA

Gonorrhoea is much more common than syphilis – 20,000 to 25,000 new cases are diagnosed in Great Britain each year. It is the third most common STD, after non-specific genital infections and thrush, but much more common than genital herpes.

More than half of gonorrhoea cases are among under 24-year-olds, with three to five times as many cases among young men as among young women. Today there are probably between 200 and 500 million new cases every year in the world.

WHAT IS GONORRHOEA?

The gonorrhoea organism is small and bean-shaped, and is passed on by sexual intercourse – oral and anal as well as vaginal. It can therefore be passed from the urethra of a man, to the cervix, urethra, throat or rectum of his partner. It can be passed to a male as well as female partner. A woman can pass it on to the urethra of her male partner during penetration.

Since the organism (gonococcus) dies very quickly outside the human body, it is virtually impossible to pass it on without sexual intercourse. So you need not worry about catching it from a lavatory seat or towel. But if you do have sexual intercourse with someone

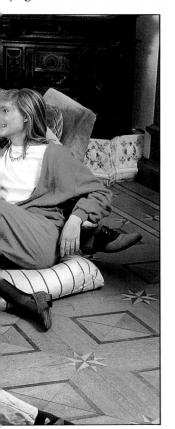

One of the most important elements in the treatment of STDs is the tracing of contacts, particularly as many women have no symptoms

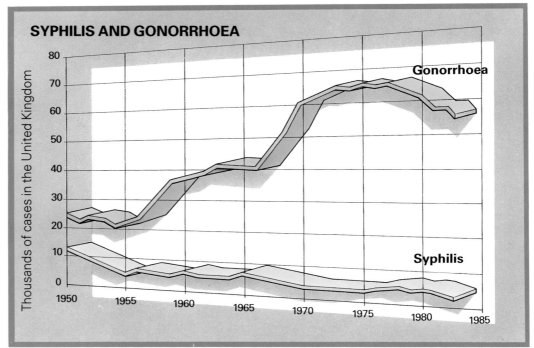

who has gonorrhoea, you have more than an even chance of catching it.

THE SYMPTOMS

The symptoms are different in men and women. While only one man in ten is symptomless, over half the women who develop the disease have no symptoms.

The first signs for a man occur between three and five days after contact with an infected partner. They start with a tingling of the man's urethra, followed by a thick, creamy-yellow discharge, which drips from the penis. At the same time there is a burning pain on passing urine.

Although at first he feels well in himself, if the infection is not treated and spreads, he may well begin to suffer from fever and headaches within ten to fourteen days. Infection can then travel to the prostate gland, the bladder, the testes or the epididymis. Scarring of the epididymis – the two long narrow tubes where sperm mature before they are ejaculated – can cause permanent sterility if both are affected.

Symptoms of gonorrhoea in a woman may include vaginal discharge or a burning feeling when passing urine. One painful complication occurs when the glands which supply secretions to keep the vagina moist become swollen and tender.

If the infection is not treated, it may spread upwards, often during menstruation, and affect the Fallopian tubes. This may happen in as many as one in ten women who contract gonorrhoea, and is accompanied by fever, headaches, and severe pelvic pain. The inflammation of the tubes, known as salpingitis, can be serious enough to need emergency hospital admission, and the resultant scarring and blocking of the tubes can lead to permanent sterility.

TREATMENT

A positive diagnosis, found by microscope examination of penile discharge, or of a smear taken from a woman's urethra, vagina or cervix, is followed by treatment with penicillin. If oral sex has taken place, a swab is taken from the throat, and if anal intercourse has occured, one is taken from the rectum.

Treatment today usually consists of one large dose of penicillin in tablet form, together with Probenecid which maintains high levels of the antibiotic in the blood stream. While treatment is taking place, it is very important to avoid alcohol and sexual contact, usually for a matter of weeks, until all signs of the infection are gone and the patient is pronounced clear.

A week following treatment, more swabs are taken and checked for gonocuccus. If none is present the man is considered cured, but a woman needs to be checked again, after her next period.

PREVENTION

For both syphilis and gonorrhora, the condom may provide a degree of protection, and it is accepted that the diaphragm or cap can protect the cervix from infection. Passing urine after sex may also help a woman to avoid gonorrhoea, although none of these measures guarantee protection.

NSU IN MEN

There were around 85,000 cases of non-specific genital infections reported in British clinics in 1989, and the numbers remain discouragingly high.

The most common non-specific infection in men is non-specific urethritis (NSU), also called non-gonococcal urethritis. Urethritis is an inflammation of the urethra. It is termed non-specific, when no particular cause (such as gonococcus which causes gonorrhoea) can be found. Although various germs may be responsible for NSU, in about half the cases an organism called chlamydia is present.

Because women have a shorther urethra than men, they seldom develop NSU itself, but the germs can infect the cervix without producing any symptoms.

When a man catches NSU, the infection usually starts about a week or two after sexual contact. He experiences pain on passing urine, and feels the need to go more often. He also has a discharge from his penis – a discharge which looks exactly like that of gonorrhoea and can only be differentiated by microscopic examination.

TREATMENT AND TRACING

A number of antibiotics can be used to treat NSU. The most commonly prescribed are tetracyclines. Tablets are taken over a period of a week or more, and during this time alcohol should be avoided. It is also important that there is no sexual contact and that sexual partners are traced as soon as possible.

A check-up is usually carried out after a week to confirm that gonorrhoea is not present, and again after a further week or so, to check that the infection is cured. If the infection is not quickly treated, the organism (usually chlamydia) may spread to other organs.

When the bladder is infected, urinating becomes very difficult and painful. If it reaches the prostrate gland there is pain in the pelvic area. The infection can spread further to produce conjunctivitis and the slow development of arthritis. The arthritis is sometimes accompanied by fever, and a general feeling of being unwell, and is known as Reiters syndrome. It is usually cured after a few months, but further attacks can lead to permanent damage to the joints if nothing is done to treat them.

GENITAL HERPES

The number of cases of genital herpes diagnosed each year is slowly rising. In Britain there are around 20,000 cases annually, which makes it the sixth most common STD. There has been a great deal written about this so-called 'new' disease. Yet the herpes virus has been around for hundreds of years, and blood tests show that over half of all adults have been infected with the virus – although most of them have no symptoms.

THE TWO TYPES

There are two types of herpes simplex virus, known as type 1 and 2. The first usually causes cold sores around the mouth and nose. Type 2 usually causes sores in the genital and anal area, but can spread to the mouth. The two types of virus are very similar and can only be told apart by tests in the laboratory.

Most people have built up antibodies to the type 1 virus by the time they are adults, although most of them will have had no symptoms. Fewer will have built up this resistance to type 2 virus in childhood and adolescence, as it is usually passed on by sexual contact.

It is known that herpes can be passed from the mouth to the genital area. When an adult is infected with the simplex 2 virus, there is about an even chance he or she will develop no symptoms.

HERPES SYMPTOMS

The first symptoms of an attack occur within seven days of genital contact. A man will feel a tingling or itching along his penis (or anus) and a woman around the vulva. Sometimes there are 'flu-like symptoms, with headache, backache or a temperature.

Very quickly small, painful, reddish bumps appear in the places where there was itching. By the next day they have become small blisters. These can be very painful, particularly during the first attack, and for the woman the whole area may become swollen so that it is difficult to pass urine. Sometimes the blisters are not visible, and go unnoticed inside the vagina or rectum.

Next, the blisters burst and leave small red ulcers that crust over and heal in a week or so. The area is infectious for about a week after the ulcers have healed, and the virus can be passed on by sexual contact, or by touching, during this time.

RECURRENT ATTACKS

For about half of those who have a first attack of herpes, it will be their last. But for the other half, recurrent attacks happen with varying frequency. What triggers this off is still uncertain and may vary from person to person. Possible triggers are:
- ☐ stress
- ☐ hormonal changes
- ☐ friction during intercourse
- ☐ sunbathing or using sunbeds
- ☐ tight clothes or nylon underwear.

MEDICAL TREATMENT

If you think you are having an attack, go to your doctor or special clinic. Diagnosis is made by taking swabs, and the results can be ready within 24 hours.

Although there is no known absolute cure, there are drugs which make the sores less painful, and one drug, acyclovir, which effectively treats the initial attack. This is usually taken by mouth, but is sometimes used as an ointment. It does not, however, seem to prevent or effectively treat future attacks – although there is some evidence that it can help ward

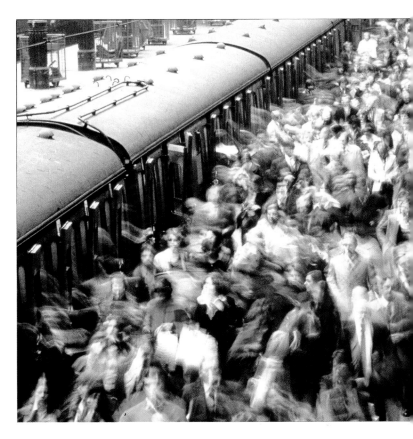

For many people the first attack of genital herpes is often the last – but other may suffer recurrent attacks. If this happens to you, look closely at your lifestyle. Is stress – even something as common as travelling in the rush hour – acting as a trigger?

them off if used immediately when an attack seem imminent.

Suggestions for relieving the painful area include:
- ☐ bathing in a salt solution
- ☐ applying an ice-pack to the sores
- ☐ sitting in a warm bath with potassium permanganate in it
- ☐ leaving sores exposed to the air as much as possible
- ☐ dabbing sores with witch-hazel or surgical spirit to dry them out.

Occasionally a woman finds urinating too painful to bear when she has an attack of herpes. She can have a catheter temporarily inserted into her bladder, or she may find relief by passing urine in a warm bath.

LIFE AFTER HERPES

Although herpes is very painful, and recurrent attacks unpleasant, it need not be the end of your sex life.

There is a very small risk of passing it on when you have not got sores, and there are many other ways of giving pleasure to each other when you do. It is a good idea to talk about it with your partner, and if you need more support, there are a number of self-help groups around that will provide it.

AIDS

The world faces a major epidemic of a disease with a hidden dimension, for the AIDS virus can be carried for years without symptoms becoming evident. Despite worldwide concerted efforts, no solution is predicted for the short term, although changes in sexual behaviour can mitigate the situation

Much of the hysteria about AIDS that is gripping the world, particularly the West, is generated by society's attitudes towards some of those groups most likely to be affected – homosexuals, bisexuals and intravenous drug users.

This has resulted in an outbreak of hysteria as devastating in its way as the disease itself, which has earned the tags of AFRAIDS and AIPS (AIDS Induced Panic Syndrome). Children have been barred from classrooms, dentists have refused to treat gay patients and cameramen have boycotted interview sessions featuring victims.

The disease itself has confounded doctors and scientists alike since it was officially recognized in July 1981 in San Francisco, and a cure is not expected in the near future, despite extensive research being carried out throughout the world.

WHY AIDS KILLS
The acronym AIDS stands for Acquired Immune Deficiency Syndrome which spells out about as much and as little as we know about the disease. It is *acquired* and not inherited; it strikes at the *immune* system, the body's natural defence against hostile invading organisms; it produces a *deficiency* in its ability to fight infection; and it is a *syndrome* – a collection of symptoms which seem to occur together and very probably have the same cause.

AIDS-RELATED DISEASE
Victims die not from AIDS itself, but from one of a host of diseases to which the human body deprived of its immune system can fall prey.

Chief among these are Kaposi's sarcoma (a rare and disfiguring skin cancer) and a type of pneumonia (*Pneumocystis carinii pneumonia*) hardly ever seen except in cases of AIDS. Together or separately, these two diseases have caused about three-quarters of the deaths of AIDS victims in both Britain and the United States of America.

UNKNOWN ORIGIN
Equally puzzling is the origin of AIDS. Many researchers believe the virus was perhaps passed from animals to humans in day-to-day contact.

Monkeys in Africa, pigs in Haiti, even sheep in Iceland have all been singled out as possible one-time hosts of the virus, but no one really knows how and why it claimed humans as its victims.

There is mounting evidence that AIDS is in fact an old disease from Africa, where the cancer Kaposi's sarcoma is thought to have been known long before the current outbreak.

AIDS IN THE USA
Wherever it came from, the disease has spread extremely rapidly over long distances in a very short

As with most living organisms, the AIDS virus must kill in order to procreate and survive. Unfortunately, its natural prey – the T4 cell – is part of the immune system. While the virus is as fragile as a soap bubble outside the human body, once it reaches the blood stream it becomes, to date, impossible to destroy

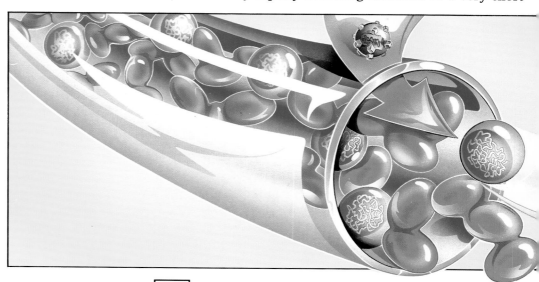

space of time. The problem is that whereas most diseased increase arithmetically (2, 4, 6, 8 and so on) AIDS increases exponentially (2, 4, 8, 16, 32), and this is what has led to the cliff-face rise in the numbers affected. In America, five cases of *Pneumocystis carinii pneumonia* in Los Angeles and 26 cases of Kaposi's sarcoma in New York and California heralded the arrival of the disease in the summer of 1981.

THREAT TO HETEROSEXUALS

By the end of October 1990, over 150,000 cases of AIDS had been officially notified in the USA and up to 95,000 deaths from the disease had been recorded. It is believed that the rapid increase in the number of cases in previous years was due to the fact that some homosexuals were considerably more promiscuous than heterosexual men or women. However, as the latest figures for gonorrhoea show that incidences within the gay community are declining – whereas heterosexual cases are still increasing – it can be assumed that homosexual promiscuity has declined. This, together with increasing awareness of safe sexual practices, has made doctors hopeful that the increase in gay AIDS cases will decline.

AIDS IN THE UK

Hot on the heels of the American outbreak of the disease came its British appearance, and although the numbers involved are far smaller, the rate of increase in the numbers of AIDS sufferers in the United Kingdom has been equally dramatic.

The first case of AIDS in the United Kingdom was reported in December 1981, with the first death, that of a 37-year-old man, on 4th July 1982. By February 1991 the number of AIDS cases reported in the UK stood at 4,354 and the number of AIDS-related deaths at 2,493.

AIDS WORLDWIDE

By 1st December 1990 the number of AIDS cases notified to the World Health Organisation (WHO) had exceeded 300,000, although WHO estimates that the true number of AIDS sufferers worldwide is far greater than this.

Russia has finally acknowledged that it does have the beginnings of an AIDS problem, but the governments of other countries, particularly those dependent on their tourist trade, are keeping quiet about the actual incidence of the disease. Undoubtedly, AIDS is no respecter of borders – cases are being identified in developing nations as in the West, in small towns and in the country, as well as in larger cities.

NOT A HOMOSEXUAL DISEASE

Although AIDS has been dubbed by some as the gay plague and has even been described as being the result of the wrath of God brought to bear on homosexuals, it is by no means exclusive to the gay pooulation, nor even the male population.

In Europe and and US, male homosexuals have made up the majority of victims to date, but other high risk groups include intravenous drug users, haemophiliacs using blood products, bisexuals and prostitutes. In the US and UK a number of sufferers are heterosexual men and women, proof of the fact that anyone who has sex is now at risk.

Outside of the western world, the concentration of AIDS in the gay population has been far less of a feature of the disease. In Central Africa, for example, where as many as one in 10 people are affected in some areas, AIDS is spreading rapidly through heterosexual contact and women are just as likely as men to fall victim to the disease, particularly prostitutes. This may be because of poor standards of hygiene in hospitals and clinics. But it may also be the result of the widespread practice of anal intercourse as a form of contraception in some African countries.

VIRUS ISOLATED

When people were first striken by AIDS, doctors were mystified and the actual cause of this deadly disease was only isolated in 1985. The culprit is a virus which

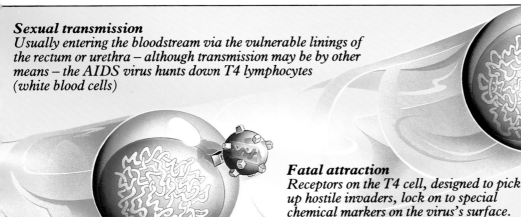

Sexual transmission
Usually entering the bloodstream via the vulnerable linings of the rectum or urethra – although transmission may be by other means – the AIDS virus hunts down T4 lymphocytes (white blood cells)

Fatal attraction
Receptors on the T4 cell, designed to pick up hostile invaders, lock on to special chemical markers on the virus's surface. Now the T4 cell will begin to release antibodies, but to no avail

THE SAFER SEX CODE
1. Only solo sex is guaranteed safe.
2. Avoid any contact with your partner's semen, bodily fluids or blood.
3. Have sex where you do not orgasm inside your partner's body, or if you feel you must do so, use a condom.
Supplied by the Terence Higgins Trust.

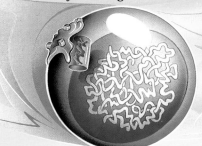
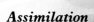

Insertion
As the antibodies begin their attack, the virus discards its outer coat. Now the core of the virus insinuates itself into the cell. Since the core contains RNA and not DNA, the cell is unaware of the danger

Assimilation
Once safely in place, the virus continues to fool its unsuspecting host by using an enzyme to change its RNA into DNA. The genetic material is treated by T4 cells as if it were its very own

attacks the very cells which protect us from infection. This rod-shaped bug has been labelled the HTLV III virus (or human T cell lymphotropic virus, Type 3) by American scientists, and LAV (lymphaedenopathy associated virus) by French scientists. They have now compromised and the virus is known as LAV-HTLV III. Since the isolation of the original virus, another, more virulent, strain of the disease has been identified and others may exist.

How the AIDS virus spreads from one person to another is still not completely understood. Scientists have isolated it in most body fluids of AIDS victims – in blood, semen and saliva. But because the virus can be isolated in a laboratory test tube does not mean that it can be passed on through contact with all these fluids. AIDS is predominantly a blood-borne disease, although semen is also a likely carrier.

What is clear is that those in normal daily contact with AIDS victims are not necessarily in danger.

ANAL TRANSMISSION
The most common method of transmission is still through anal intercourse. The reason why anal intercourse allows the virus to cross over from one host to another is because the membranes of the rectum are much more delicate than those of the vagina, and hence far more likely to tear and bleed.

Unlike the vagina, the walls of the rectum allow fluids to pass through into the blood stream, so viruses from contaminated sperm could enter another person's body in this way.

There are two other ways in which the virus might be spread by blood to blood contact; by exchanging and using infected needles, a common practice among intravenous drug users; and by transfusing contaminated blood or blood products.

OTHERS AT RISK
Haemophiliacs have found themselves in a high risk group because of their treatment with the blood clotting agent, Factor VIII.

However, these two routes of transmission – blood transfusions and contaminated Factor VIII – should have been blocked by the introduction of tests for all blood donors and of heat-treating all blood to kill off any AIDS viruses present. These measures have been mandatory in the UK since September 1985.

MANY SYMPTOMS
When they do develop, the symptoms of AIDS are those of an array of diseases to which the immune deficient victim has fallen prey, making it difficult to tell whether someone actually has the disease. These include swollen glands in the neck, armpit or groin, weight loss, high fever and night sweats, diarrhoea and persistent coughs or shortness of breath.

There may also be skin changes with pink or purple flattish blotches or bumps occuring on or under the skin, inside the mouth, nose, eyelids or rectum or blemishes in the mouth.

Where any of these symptoms occur alone, or even in twos and threes, it is extremely unlikely that AIDS will be found to be the cause, and because the fear of AIDS can be almost as debilitating as the disease itself, it is important to seek medical advice.

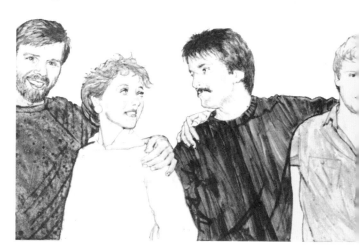

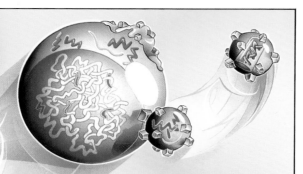

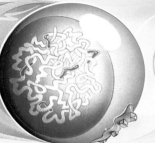

ll death
e AIDS DNA may lie hidden for up to
e years within the T4 chromosomes.
nw and why it becomes activated remains
nystery – but when it does, the cell begins
make copies of the virus and dies

DNA – *found only within the cell nucleus, it stores the genetic code and can (uniquely) replicate itself*
RNA – *found throughout the cell, it can act as a messenger for DNA in synthesizing the protein chains that are part of the human body*

COMPLETE CURE NOT YET IN SIGHT

As yet, the prospects for the prevention and cure of AIDS look none too hopeful.

No known cure has yet been found for the disease and the best that can be done, medically, for victims is to help alleviate the symptoms. Nor is there any effective vaccine at present, and according to scientists there is no chance of there being one in the near future.

The virus probably has several different forms, each capable of mutating (changing), which makes the development of a vaccine difficult. Many of the drugs currently being tested as possible cures for AIDS are aimed at stopping the virus reproducing after it has entered the body, but progress is slow. According to a report in the New England Journal of Medicine, doctors have isolated the virus in the brain and spinal fluid from AIDS sufferers. The implications are that the virus 'hides' in the brain – and this could make

One of the most distressing facts about the AIDS virus is that it can lie undetected for some years before the carrier shows any symptoms. Thus the virus can be passed unwittingly from one person to another, as there is no obvious way of telling who is infected during this dormant period

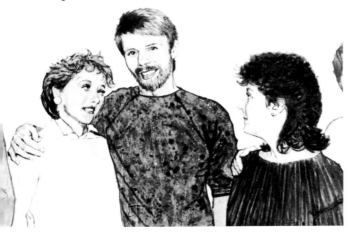

eradication difficult, though probably not impossible.

Despite the anxiety among health care workers, and those involved in caring for AIDS victims, their chances of contracting the disease themselves seem remote. Apart from a handful of accidental contamination with the AIDS virus caused by syringe injuries, mainly in the USA, there have been no known cases of the disease being contracted at work by doctors or nurses.

It is, however, known that an infected mother can pass on AIDS to her unborn child, possibly through the placenta or else during the actual birth when blood is lost by the mother.

VIRUS NOT NECESSARILY FATAL

As yet there is no test which shows categorically whether a person has AIDS. Anyone who has come into contact with the virus will make antibodies to it, and will show up as 'antibody positive'.

But although the presence of antibodies gives no protection against the disease, only 5–10 per cent of those who are found to have HIV antibodies in the blood go on to develop a fatal case of AIDS.

Some will develop milder, less life-threatening infections, and a sizeable number may develop no obvious symptoms at all.

AIDS CARRIERS

Exactly what makes one person develop the disease while others remain unaffected is not known exactly, but carriers – those who have antibodies without symptoms – will still be capable of passing the virus to others, who in turn will stand much the same chance of developing AIDS.

The other worrying problem about AIDS is that symptoms make take anything from two, possibly as long as seven, years to emerge, which means that sufferers may unwittingly be infecting a large number of other people before realizing they have the disease. With this in mind, many countries worldwide have programmes aimed at preventing the spread of AIDS.

INDEX

A

Afterplay 120
  sexual problems, helping with 163
AIDS
  anal transmission of 188
  carriers 189
  cure for 189
  diseases related to 186
  fatal, not necessarily 189
  gay population, in 187
  heterosexuals, threat to 187
  hysteria about 186
  meaning 186
  origin of 186
  safe sex code 187
  symptoms of 188
  transmission of 188
  UK, in 187
  USA, in 186, 187
  virus, 187, 188
  worldwide 187
Anal stimulators 133, 139
Armpits
  using in lovemaking 89

B

Bath
  love-making in 17, 87
  sensual 188
Bathing together 12
Bathroom
  love-making in 17
Bedroom
  dressing for 27, 28
  sexier, making 19
Body hair 20, 21
Bondage 87
Books, sexy 135
Brassiere, invention of 24
Breasts
  arousal, and 32–34
  big-breasted women 30, 31
  breastplay 34
  excitement phase 33
  girls' ambivalent attitude to 31
  ideal 31
  influences on 31
  obsession with 30
  orgasm, effect of 33
  part of sex-appeal, as 31
  plateau phase 33
  pleasure, use in increasing 34
  resolution phase 33
  self-exploration 31, 32
  size and sensitivity 32
  use to excite 34, 35
  using in lovemaking 89
Bust enlargement creams 134

C

Caressing, intimate 53
Clitoral stimulators 135, 138
Clothes
  black underwear 28
  butch he-man look 29
  erotic potential 27
  fantasy 25
  femme fatale look 29
  French tart look 29
  frilly underwear 28
  Latin lover look 29
  leather and latex 24, 28
  legs, revealing 26
  little boy lost 29
  partner's likes and dislikes, getting to know 28
  plumage, as 24
  pop star look 29
  professional woman look 28
  sensitive poet look 29
  servant look 28
  sexually attractive 25, 26
  sexually stimulating 24
  sexy schoolgirl look 28
  sexy underwear 135, 138
  sportsman look 29
  toff look 29
  tomboy look 28
Codpiece 24
Contraception
  barrier methods 179, 180
  choice, sharing 176
  coil 178–180
  information about 176
  IUD 178–180
  longer-acting 178
  male pills 178
  methods and effectiveness 177
  mini-Pill, the 178
  Pill, the 177
  post-coital IUD 181
  post-coital Pill 181
  safe period methods 180, 181
  spontaneous sex, for 85
  sterilization 181
  turn-on, as 89
Courtship games 101

D

Daydreaming, sexual 40
Declining sex
  courtship behaviour, return to 164, 165
  improving 164, 165
  oral lovemaking, using 165–168
  reasons for 164
  variety, using 168, 169
Dildoes, using 137, 138
Dressing 12
  attract, to 25, 26
  bedroom, for 27, 28
  image, projecting 27
  imaginative sex, for 87
  romantic 116
  seduction, for 107
  sex, for 24–29
  sexuality, expressing 26, 27
  spontaneous sex, for 85
  undress, to 28, 29

E

Erections
  problems, fantasy helping with 47

F

Feet 89
Female fantasies
  complications 41
  encouragement of, 70
  explanation of 39–41
  foreplay, and 39
  hidden 36, 37
  men's attitude to 40
  orgasm, and 39
  same-sex 39
  sexual daydreaming 40
  subject-matter of 37–39
  talking about 41
  time for 39
Fetishes
  fantasy, and 47
  magical powers, having 149
  males, predominant in 149
  meaning 148
  morality, and 149
  narrow view 149
  restrictions 148
  rubber 152
  starting 148
  types of 149
  underwear 150, 151
Food
  imaginative sex, use in 87, 88
Foreplay
  fantasy, and 39
  flagging sex life, reviving 167
  imaginative 51
  massage 11, 12
  quality of 69
  seduction, during 101, 102
  sexual problems, helping with 163

G

G spot
  his, massaging 65
  men's 127
  orgasm 57, 127
  touching 63
Genital herpes 184, 185
Genitals
  washing 20
Gonorrhoea 183, 184
Group sex
  changing partners 153
  comparison, leading to 157
  dangers of 154
  desire for, practical solutions 155
  dissatisfaction in 157
  fantasies 157
  films of 154
  jealousy 154
  learning through watching 154
  new experience, as 153
  partner, sharing 157
  Sandstone experiment 153, 154
  two women, image of 155, 157

H

Holiday, sex on 84
Hygiene
  preparation for lovemaking, and 19, 20

I

Ideal form 25, 26
Imaginative sex
  armpits, using 89
  bathing or swimming, during 87
  bondage 87
  breaking routines 83
  breasts, using 89
  contraception, using 89
  dressing up 87
  feet, using 89
  food, use of 87, 88
  holiday, on 84
  mirrors, using 88
  need for 82, 83
  photographs, use of 88
  rear entry 89
  sleep, in 86
  spontaneous 84, 85
  waking up, on 86, 87

K

Kitchen
  love-making in 16

L

Local anaesthetic
  creams and sprays 134
Lounge
  love-making in 14–16
Love dolls 133, 139
Lovemaking
  afternoon, in 12
  atmosphere for 51
  bathroom, in 17
  dressing and undressing 12
  early morning 11, 12
  evening, in 13
  fire, in front of 14
  getting in the mood for 21
  hygiene and preparation 19, 20
  kitchen, in 16
  lounge, in 14–16
  lunchtime, at 12
  making time for 18, 19
  milestone 50
  movement in 71, 90–95
  number of times of 172
  place for 14–17, 83
  props for 129
  rhythm and timing, importance of 57
  right mood for 51
  romantic 118–121
  romantic places for 117
  routine 11, 50, 82
  semi-public places, in 83, 84
  sport, after 84, 87
  stairs, on 16, 17
  surprise 169
  time for 11–14
  time of month for 18
  weekdays, during 11
Lubricants 88, 133, 139

M

Male fantasies
  clinical uses of 47
  compliant partners, about 45, 46
  creative 44
  erection problems, helping with 47
  explanation of 46
  fetishism, and 47
  learning process, in 43
  persistent images 43
  private 43
  subject-matter of 43, 44
  use of 46
Male masturbation aids 132, 139
Massage
  early morning 11, 12
  romantic 120
  seduction, during 111
  sensual, learning 22, 23
Masturbation
  aids 132, 139
  encouragement of 70
  her to him 63
  Him to her 61–63
  learning through 60

movement 90, 91
oil, using 53, 55, 62, 63
purpose of 160
right position for 60
special needs, being aware of 61
timing 59, 60
uses of 58, 59
vagina, exploration of 62, 63, 21, 22
Memorable sex 51
Menstruation
lovemaking during 21, 88
Mini-Pill, the 177
Mirrors 88
Movement
full stroke, positions permitting 92
indirect 91
little, position permitting 94
lovemaking, during 71, 91–95
masturbation, in 90, 91
men, by 92
positions for woman 94
thrusting 95
woman, by 91, 92

N

Non-specific urethritis 184

O

Oil, using 53, 55, 62, 63
Oral sex 12
flagging sex life, reviving 165–168
her, for 74–77
him, for 64, 65, 78–81
mutual 55, 56
non-genital 74, 75
orgasm, improving 127, 128
positions for 65
romantic 119, 120
seduction during 112
sexual problems, helping with 162
timing 59, 60
tips for 74, 78
uses of 58, 59
variations 75, 76, 79, 80
vibrator, use with 64
Orgasm
coming too soon 160, 161
difficulty in achieving 161, 162
early, advantage of 68, 72
failure to achieve 73
familiarity, and 123, 124
fantasy, and 39
female lead 71, 73
G spot 57, 127
improving 124
intercourse, alternatives to 129
male lead 68–71
man, speeding up 73
new techniques, using 124
needs, anticipating 57
oral sex, with 127, 128
pelvic muscles, using 92
sexual techniques, importance of 123
simultaneous 67–73
taking the lead 67, 68
teasing 52, 53
timing 66
variation in 122, 123
vibrator, using 124–126, 137
woman taking control 126, 127
69 position, in 55

P

Pelvic muscles, using 92

Penile rings 134, 139
Penile toys 134
Pheromone sprays 135
Photographs 88
Pill, the 177
Pornography 88

Q

Quickie sex 85

R

Romance
acting romantically 115–117
afterplay 120
bath, sensual 118
consideration 116
dressing up 116
her to him loving 120, 121
him to her loving 117–120
importance of 115
kissing and cuddling 117
loss of 115
male, romantic 114
massage, use of 120
places for making love 117
preparation for lovemaking 117
recipient of 115
restoration of 115
sharing activities 116
surprise, use of 115
touching 116
women, and 114, 115
Routine sex life 11
Rubber fetish 152

S

Security, effect on sex life 164
Seduction of husband
aftermath 112
arousal 109
atmosphere for 108
bath, masturbation in 109
dressing for 107
familiarity, using 106, 107
kissing and caressing 111
making love 112
massage 111
meal 109
oral sex 112
preparation for 107, 108
tactics 107
video, watching 109
Seduction of wife
aftermath 104
attention, giving 99
clothes, removing 101
courtship games 101
dancing together 101
dinner, intimate 99
foreplay 101, 102
long-term partner, of 96
making love 104
preparation for 96
relaxation 96, 99
vibrator, using 102
warm-up to 96
Semi-public places
lovemaking in 83, 84
Sex aids 21
anal stimulators 133, 139
books 135
clitoral stimulators 135, 138
creams, sprays and potions, 134, 135
dildoes 132, 137, 138
finger covers 135
love dolls 133, 139
love eggs 135, 136
lubricants 133, 139

male masturbation aids 132, 139
penile rings 134, 139
penile toys 134
sexy underwear 135, 138
sheaths 133, 138
using 136–139
vaginal stimulators 139
vibrators, see Vibrators
videos 135
Sex drive, variation in 122, 123
Sex hormones
peak time for 12
Sex toys 21, 135
Sexual activity
early 170, 171
fifties, in 172, 174
forties, in 171, 172, 174
golden rules 174, 175
sixties, in 172, 174, 175
thirties, in 171–174
twenties, in 171–173
Sexual behaviour 52
Sexual diseases
AIDS, see AIDS
genital herpes 184, 185
gonorrhoea 183, 184
non-specific urethritis 184
persons suffering from 182
syphilis 182, 183
Sexual peak, time of 170
Sexual positions
changing 56
full penetration but little movement, permitting 92, 94
full stroke movement, permitting 92
little movement, for 94
missionary 71
new, trying 168
oral sex, for 65
rear entry 71, 89, 129
romantic 119, 121
side entry 71
woman on top 72, 73
woman, for movement of 94
"69" 55, 167, 168
Sexual problems
coming too soon 160, 161
couples, sorted out between 159
failure to come 161, 162
female myths 159
helping, her for him 159–162
helping, him for her 162, 163
male worries 158
performance, myth of 158, 159
pressure, taking of 160
squeeze technique 160
Sexual rut, falling into 82
Sheaths 133, 138
Showering together 12
Showers
oral sex in 17
sex in 87
Sleeping, sex during 86
Sofa, love-making on 14–16
Spontaneous sex 84, 85
dressing for 85
preparation for 85
Sport, making love after 84, 87
Squeeze technique 160
Stairs, love-making on 16, 17
Swimming pool, sex in 87
Syphilis 182, 183

T

Time for sex 11–14

U

Underwear
fetishes 150, 151

sexy 28, 135, 138

V

Vaginal stimulators 139
Vibrator
basic model 132
creative use of 10
genitals, using on 136, 137
men using 137
oral sex, use with 64
orgasm, improving 137
seduction, suing during 102
sex aid, as 132
using 54, 124–146, 136
Videos
action 147
anticipation in 147
body care for 145
camera, working 143
contract 142
editing 146
lighting 143
location 142, 143
making 140–147
movements 147
outdoors, shooting 144
pornographic 157
script, sticking to 145
setting up camera 140
sexy 135
shooting 145
story-line 141, 142
striptease 145
test shots 140
viewing 147
wardrobe and props 145
zooming 140

W

Waking up
sex on, 86, 87

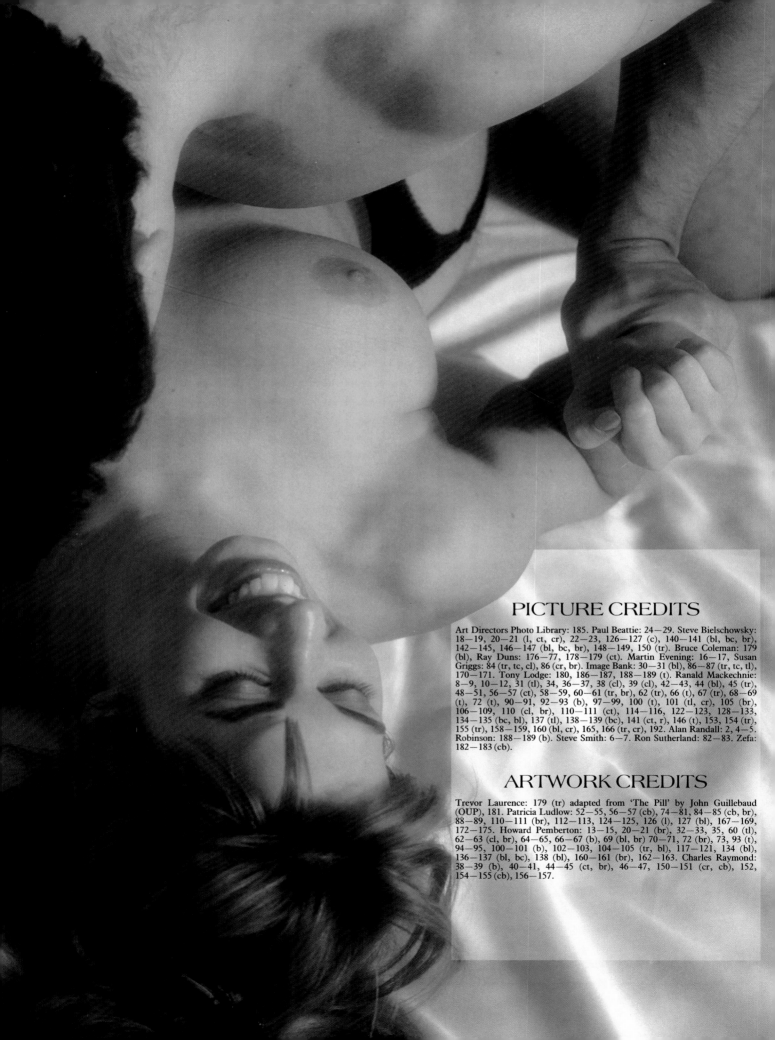

PICTURE CREDITS

Art Directors Photo Library: 185. Paul Beattie: 24—29. Steve Bielschowsky:
18—19, 20—21 (l, ct, cr), 22—23, 126—127 (c), 140—141 (bl, bc, br),
142—145, 146—147 (bl, bc, br), 148—149, 150 (tr). Bruce Coleman: 179
(bl), Ray Duns: 176—77, 178—179 (ct). Martin Evening: 16—17, Susan
Griggs: 84 (tr, tc, cl), 86 (cr, br). Image Bank: 30—31 (bl), 86—87 (tr, tc, tl),
170—171. Tony Lodge: 180, 186—187, 188—189 (t). Ranald Mackechnie:
8—9, 10—12, 31 (tl), 34, 36—37, 38 (cl), 39 (cl), 42—43, 44 (bl), 45 (tr),
48—51, 56—57 (ct), 58—59, 60—61 (tr, br), 62 (tr), 66 (t), 67 (tr), 68—69
(t), 72 (t), 90—91, 92—93 (b), 97—99, 100 (t), 101 (tl, cr), 105 (br),
106—109, 110 (cl, br), 110—111 (ct), 114—116, 122—123, 128—133,
134—135 (bc, bl), 137 (tl), 138—139 (bc), 141 (ct, r), 146 (t), 153, 154 (tr),
155 (tr), 158—159, 160 (bl, cr), 165, 166 (tr, cr), 192. Alan Randall: 2, 4—5.
Robinson: 188—189 (b). Steve Smith: 6—7. Ron Sutherland: 82—83. Zefa:
182—183 (cb).

ARTWORK CREDITS

Trevor Laurence: 179 (tr) adapted from 'The Pill' by John Guillebaud
(OUP), 181. Patricia Ludlow: 52—55, 56—57 (cb), 74—81, 84—85 (cb, br),
88—89, 110—111 (br), 112—113, 124—125, 126 (l), 127 (bl), 167—169,
172—175. Howard Pemberton: 13—15, 20—21 (br), 32—33, 35, 60 (tl),
62—63 (cl, br), 64—65, 66—67 (b), 69 (bl, br) 70—71, 72 (br), 73, 93 (t),
94—95, 100—101 (b), 102—103, 104—105 (tr, bl), 117—121, 134 (bl),
136—137 (bl, bc), 138 (bl), 160—161 (br), 162—163. Charles Raymond:
38—39 (b), 40—41, 44—45 (ct, br), 46—47, 150—151 (cr, cb), 152,
154—155 (cb), 156—157.